Antiarrhythmic Drugs

A Practical Guide

Antiarrhythmic Drugs

A Practical Guide

Richard N. Fogoros, M.D.

Professor of Medicine
MCP–Hahnemann School of Medicine
Allegheny University of the Health Sciences
Director, Clinical Electrophysiology
Allegheny General Hospital
Pittsburgh, Pennsylvania

b

Blackwell Science

Blackwell Science
Editorial offices:
350 Main Street, Malden, Massachusetts
02148, USA
Osney Mead, Oxford OX2 0E1, England
25 John Street, London WC1N 2BL,
England
23 Ainslie Place, Edinburgh EH3 6AJ,
Scotland
54 University Street, Carlton, Victoria
3053, Australia
Other Editorial Offices:
Arnettee Blackwell SA, 224, Boulevard
Saint Germain, 75007 Paris, France
Blackwell Wissenschafts-Verlag GmbH
Kurfürstendamm 57, 10707 Berlin,
Germany
Zehetnergasse 6, A-1140 Vienna, Austria

Acquisitions: Chris Davis
Production: Ellen Samia
Manufacturing: Lisa Flanagan
Typeset by Best-Set Typesetters Ltd.
Printed and bound by Capital City Press, Inc.
© 1997 by Blackwell Science, Inc.
Printed in the United States of America

97 98 99 00 5 4 3 2 1

The Blackwell Science logo is a trade mark
of Blackwell Science Ltd., registered at the
United Kingdom Trade Marks Registry

DISTRIBUTORS:
USA
  Blackwell Science, Inc.
  350 Main Street
  Malden, Massachusetts 02148
  (*Telephone orders*: 800-215-1000 or
                        617-388-8250;
      Fax orders: 617-388-8270)

Canada
  Copp Clark Professional
  200 Adelaide Street, West, 3rd Floor
  Toronto, Ontario M5H 1W7
  (*Telephone orders*: 416-597-1616
                       1-800-815-9417
      Fax orders: 416-597-1617

Australia
  Blackwell Science Pty., Ltd.
  54 University Street
  Carlton, Victoria 3053
  (*Telephone orders*: 03-9347-0300;
      Fax orders: 03-9349-3016)

Outside North America and Australia
  Blackwell Science, Ltd.
  c/o Marston Book Services, Ltd.
  P.O. Box 269
  Abingdon
  Oxon OX14 4YN
  England
  (*Telephone orders*: 44-01235-465500;
      Fax orders: 44-01235-465555)

Library of Congress
Cataloging-in-Publication Data

Fogoros, Richard N.
    Antiarrhythmic drugs: a practical
  guide/Richard N. Fogoros.
        p.   cm.
    Includes bibliographical references and
  index.
    ISBN 0-86542-124-2 (pbk.)
    1. Myocardial depressants.
    2. Arrhythmia—Chemotherapy.
    I. Title
    [DNLM: 1. Anti-Arrhythmia Agents.
    2. Arrhythmia—drug therapy.
    QV 150 F656a   1996]
    RM347.F64   1996
    616.1′28061—dc21
    DNLM/DLC
    for Library of Congress   96-45956
                                          CIP

Contents

Preface

Physicians once found it convenient to think of cardiac arrhythmias as a sort of "itch" of the heart and of antiarrhythmic drugs as a soothing balm that, applied in sufficient quantities, would relieve the itch. During the past 3 decades, however, pioneering work has begun to reveal the complexities of cardiac arrhythmias and the drugs used to treat them. To the dismay of most reasonable people, the old, convenient viewpoint has proven false.

As is often the case when new knowledge destroys old assumptions, complacence has been replaced by anxiety; the appropriate use of antiarrhythmic drugs has become one of the more difficult and contentious problems in the practice of medicine. Controversies about which of the many antiarrhythmic drugs to use, how to use them, or even whether to use them are sources of apparently eternal (and often rancorous) debate among electrophysiologists. Although such disputes are invigorating to the experts (inasmuch as they serve to stimulate research and publication, not to mention a demand for visiting lecturers), the resultant uncertainty is frustrating to the nonexpert.

This book is intended for nonexperts—the practitioners, trainees, and students—who are often charged with sorting through the controversies and the uncertainties to make decisions regarding actual patients with cardiac arrhythmias. The book attempts to set out a framework for understanding antiarrhythmic drugs: how they work, what they actually do to improve (or worsen) the cardiac rhythm, and the factors one must consider in deciding when and how to use them. Such a framework, it is hoped, will not only serve as a guidepost in making clinical decisions on the use of these drugs, but also will provide a basis for interpreting new information as it is added to the divergent and contradictory medical literature on the subject.

The book is divided into three parts. Part I is an introduction to basic principles—the mechanisms of cardiac arrhythmias and how antiarrhythmic drugs work. Part II discusses the clinically relevant features of the drugs themselves. Part III draws on the basic information to explore the treatment of specific cardiac arrhythmias and emphasizes the major, continuing controversies regarding drug therapy of arrhythmias.

Throughout the book, basic principles are emphasized. Accordingly, when a choice has had to be made between simplicity and complexity, simplicity has prevailed in almost every case. The author recognizes that some colleagues may not agree with an approach that risks oversimplification of an inherently complex topic. It is an approach, however, that reflects a deep-seated belief—by keeping the basics simple, the specifics (clinical cases, scientific reports) can be more readily weighed, categorized, absorbed, and implemented.

R.N.F.

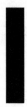

Basic Principles

Mechanisms of Cardiac Tachyarrhythmias

Using antiarrhythmic drugs appropriately is difficult. Their use is likely to be impossible unless one has a firm grasp of the basic mechanisms of cardiac tachyarrhythmias and the basic concepts of how antiarrhythmic drugs work. Part I of this book covers the basics. In Chapter 1 the normal electrical system of the heart is described, and the mechanisms and clinical features of the major cardiac tachyarrhythmias are considered. Chapter 2 examines the principles of how antiarrhythmic drugs affect arrhythmias.

THE ELECTRICAL SYSTEM OF THE HEART

On a very fundamental level, the heart is an electrical organ. The electrical signals generated by the heart not only cause muscle contraction (by controlling the flux of calcium ions across the cardiac cell membrane) but also organize the sequence of muscle contraction with each heartbeat, thus optimizing the pumping action of the heart. In addition, and more pertinent to the subject of this book, the pattern and timing of the cardiac electrical signals determine the heart rhythm. Thus, a well-functioning electrical system is vital for adequate cardiac performance.

Anatomy

The cardiac electrical impulse originates in the sinoatrial (SA) node, high in the right atrium near the superior vena cava (Figure 1.1). From the SA node the impulse spreads radially across both atria. When it reaches the atrioventricular (AV) groove, the impulse encounters the fibrous "skeleton" of the heart, which separates the atria from the ventricles. The fibrous skeleton is electrically inert,

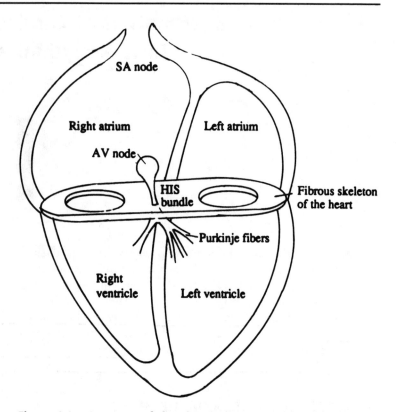

Figure 1.1. Anatomy of the electrical system of the heart.

and therefore stops the electrical impulse. The only way for the impulse to cross over to the ventricular side is by means of the specialized AV conducting tissues—the AV node and the His-Purkinje system.

The AV node conducts electricity slowly; when the electrical impulse enters the AV node, its passage is delayed. The delay is reflected in the PR interval on the surface electrocardiogram (ECG). Leaving the AV node, the electrical impulse enters the His bundle, the most proximal part of the rapidly conducting His-Purkinje system. The His bundle penetrates the fibrous skeleton and delivers the impulse to the ventricular side of the AV groove.

Once on the ventricular side, the electrical impulse follows the His-Purkinje system as it divides first into the right and left bundle branches, then into the Purkinje fibers. The Purkinje fibers speed the impulse to the furthermost reaches of the ventricular myocardium. In this way, the electrical impulse is rapidly distributed throughout the ventricles.

The heart's electrical system thus organizes the sequence of myocardial contraction with each heartbeat—as the electrical impulse spreads across the atria, the atria contract. The delay provided by the AV node allows complete emptying of the atria before the electrical impulse reaches the ventricles. Once the electrical impulse leaves the AV node, it is distributed rapidly throughout the ventricular muscle by the Purkinje fibers, thus providing brisk and orderly ventricular contraction.

Cardiac Action Potential

The electrical impulse of the heart is actually the summation of thousands of tiny electrical currents generated by thousands of individual cardiac cells. The electrical activity of an individual cardiac cell is described by the cardiac action potential (Figure 1.2). The action potential is inherently complex and nonintuitive. Fortunately, for our purposes, the few things one needs to know about the action potential are reasonably simple to understand.

The inside of every living cell has a negative electrical charge. The voltage difference across the cell membrane (normally −80 to −90 mV) is called the *transmembrane potential* and is the result of an accumulation of negatively charged molecules within the cell. The transmembrane potential remains fixed throughout the lives of most living cells.

However, some cells—notably, cardiac cells—are *excitable*. When excitable cells are stimulated in just the right way, tiny channels in the cell membrane open and close, which allows electrically charged particles—ions—to pass back and forth across the membrane. The movement of electrical current across the cell membrane occurs in a very stereotypic pattern and leads to a patterned sequence of changes in the transmembrane potential. When the stereotypic changes in voltage are graphed against time, the result is the cardiac action potential.

Although the cardiac action potential is classically divided into five phases (named, somewhat perversely, phases 0 through 4), it is most helpful to consider the action potential in terms of three general phases: depolarization, repolarization, and the resting phase.

Depolarization: The depolarization phase of the action potential, phase 0, occurs when the rapid sodium channels in the cell membrane are stimulated to open, which allows positively charged

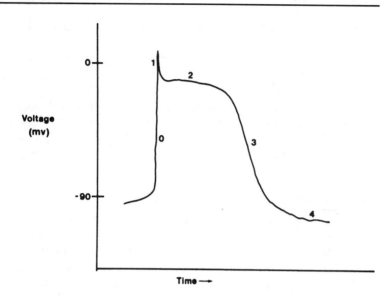

Voltage (mv)

0

-90

Time →

Figure 1.2. Cardiac action potential. Numbers on the curve indicate phases.

sodium ions to rush into the cell. The sudden influx of positive ions causes a voltage spike—a rapid, positively directed change in the transmembrane potential. The voltage spike, called *depolarization*, accounts for the heart's electrical impulse; phase 0 is when the action of the action potential occurs.

The sodium channels that allow the rapid depolarization are *voltage dependent;* that is, they open when the cell's resting transmembrane potential reaches a certain threshold voltage. The event that raises a cell's transmembrane potential to threshold voltage is most often the depolarization of a nearby cardiac cell. Thus, the depolarization of one cell leads to depolarization of adjacent cells; once a cardiac cell is depolarized, a wave of depolarization (the electrical impulse) tends to spread across the heart, cell by cell.

Further, the speed at which one cell is depolarized (represented by the slope of phase 0 of the action potential) determines how quickly the next cell is stimulated to depolarize. This sequence thus determines the speed at which the electrical impulse is propagated. If one changes the slope of phase 0, one changes conduction velocity; the faster the depolarization of the cardiac cells, the faster an electrical impulse moves across the heart.

Repolarization: If one fires a Colt 45, one cannot fire it again until it is recocked. Similarly, once a cell is depolarized, it cannot be depolarized again until the ionic fluxes that occur during depolarization are reversed. The process of getting the ions back to where they started is called *repolarization*. Repolarization corresponds to phases 1 through 3 (i.e., the width) of the action potential. Because the cell is refractory to depolarization until after it is repolarized, the time from the end of phase 0 to late in phase 3 is called the *refractory period* of the cell. The duration of the action potential thus determines the refractory period; if one does something to change the duration of the action potential, one also changes the refractory period.

The repolarization of cardiac cells is complex and incompletely understood. Repolarization begins rapidly (phase 1), but the process is almost immediately interrupted by a plateau phase (phase 2), which is unique to cardiac cells (e.g., it is not seen in nerve cells). Phase 2 is mediated by the slow calcium channels, which allow positively charged calcium ions to enter the cell slowly and thus interrupt repolarization and prolong the duration of the action potential.

The most important ionic shift during repolarization is the outward flow of positively charged potassium ions, which has the effect of returning the action potential toward its baseline, negatively polarized state. At least six different potassium "currents" have been identified; they operate at different times during the action potential and are modulated by different factors (including voltage, calcium ions, muscarinic receptors, acetylcholine, and adenosine triphosphate) under different circumstances.

Dumping sodium and calcium ions into a cardiac cell to depolarize it and then draining potassium ions out of the cell to repolarize it may return the transmembrane *voltage* to baseline levels, but these actions do not return the cell *chemistry* to the baseline state. Various poorly characterized mechanisms are called on to rectify remaining chemical imbalances (the most important of which is the sodium–potassium pump). Although depolarization seems fairly straightforward, attempting to understand repolarization quickly leads to a maze of seemingly conflicting channels, gates, receptors, and pumps (which only a basic electrophysiologist could love).

Fortunately, the essential features of repolarization are relatively simple: (1) repolarization returns the cardiac action potential to the resting transmembrane potential; (2) this process takes time;

7

③ the time, roughly corresponding to the width of the action potential, is the refractory period of cardiac tissue; ④ depolarization mainly depends on sodium channels, and repolarization mainly depends on potassium channels.

The Resting Phase: For most cardiac cells the *resting phase* (the period of time between two action potentials, corresponding to phase 4) is quiescent; there is no net movement of ions across the cell membrane.

For some cells and in some circumstances, however, the so-called resting phase is not quiescent. In these cases there is leakage of ions back and forth across the cell membrane during phase 4 in such a way as to cause a gradual increase in transmembrane potential (Figure 1.3). When the transmembrane potential reaches the threshold voltage, the appropriate channels are engaged and the cell is depolarized (since, as noted, the channels mediating depolarization are voltage dependent). Depolarization, in turn, stimulates nearby cells to depolarize, and the resultant spontaneously generated electrical impulse is then propagated across the heart. This phase 4 activity, which leads to spontaneous depolarization, is called automaticity.

Automaticity is the mechanism by which the normal heart rhythm is generated. Cells in the SA node—the pacemaker of the heart—normally have the fastest phase 4 activity. If for any reason the automaticity of the SA node fails, secondary pacemaker cells (often located in the AV junction) usually take over the pacemaker

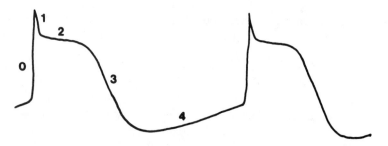

Figure 1.3. Automaticity curve. In some cardiac cells, leakage of ions across the cell membrane during phase 4 causes a gradual, positively directed change in the transmembrane voltage. When the transmembrane voltage becomes sufficiently positive, the appropriate channels are automatically activated to generate another action potential. Numbers on the curve indicate phases.

function of the heart, but they do so at a slower rate because their phase 4 activity is slower.

Localized Variations

Two localized differences in the heart's electrical system are important in understanding cardiac arrhythmias: differences in the action potential and differences in autonomic innervation.

Localized Differences in the Action Potential: The cardiac action potential does not have the same shape in every cardiac cell. The action potential shown in Figure 1.2, for instance, is a typical Purkinje fiber action potential. Figure 1.4 shows the differences in shape among the representative action potentials from several key locations of the heart. The action potentials that differ most radically from the Purkinje fiber model are found in the SA node and the AV node. Notice the slow depolarization phases (phase 0) in the action potentials. Slow depolarization occurs because the SA nodal and AV nodal tissues lack active rapid sodium channels. The SA and AV nodes are thought to depend entirely on the slow calcium channel for depolarization. Because the speed of depolarization (the slope of phase 0) determines conduction velocity, the SA and AV nodes conduct electrical impulses slowly.

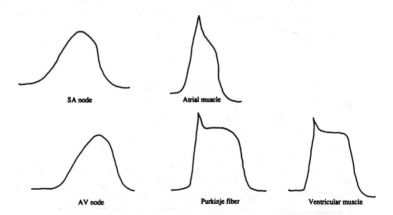

Figure 1.4. Localized differences in cardiac action potential. Action potentials generated in different areas of the heart have different shapes because different electrophysiologic properties (i.e., conduction velocity, refractoriness, and automaticity) are seen in various tissues within the heart.

Localized Differences in Autonomic Innervation: In general, an increase in sympathetic tone causes enhanced automaticity (pacemaker cells fire more rapidly), increased conduction velocity (electrical impulses spread more rapidly), and decreased refractory periods (cells are ready for repeated depolarizations more quickly). Parasympathetic tone has the opposite effect (depressed automaticity, decreased conduction velocity, and increased refractory periods).

Both sympathetic and sympathetic fibers richly supply the SA and AV nodes. In the remainder of the heart's electrical system, although sympathetic innervation is reasonably abundant, parasympathetic innervation is sparse. Thus, changes in parasympathetic tone have a relatively greater effect on the SA nodal and AV nodal tissues than they do on other tissues of the heart.

Relationship Between Action Potential and Surface Electrocardiogram

The cardiac action potential represents the electrical activity of a single cardiac cell. The surface ECG reflects the electrical activity of the entire heart. Essentially, the ECG represents the summation of all action potentials of all cardiac cells. Consequently, the information one gleans from the surface ECG derives from the characteristics of the action potential (Figure 1.5).

In most of the heart, the depolarization phase is essentially instantaneous (occurring in 1 to 3 msec) and occurs sequentially from cell to cell. Thus, the instantaneous wave of depolarization can be followed across the heart by studying the ECG. The P wave represents the depolarization front as it traverses the atria; the QRS complex represents the wave of depolarization as it spreads across the ventricles. Because depolarization is relatively instantaneous, the P wave and the QRS complex yield specific directional information. Changes in the spread of the electrical impulse, such as those that occur in bundle branch block or a transmural myocardial infarction, can be readily discerned.

In contrast, the repolarization phase of the action potential is not instantaneous; indeed, repolarization has significant duration, lasting hundreds of times longer than depolarization. Thus, although depolarization occurs from cell to cell sequentially, repolarization of the cells overlaps; all the repolarizations can be thought of as occurring simultaneously. For this reason, the ST segment and the T wave (the portions of the surface ECG that reflect ventricular repolarization) give very little directional infor-

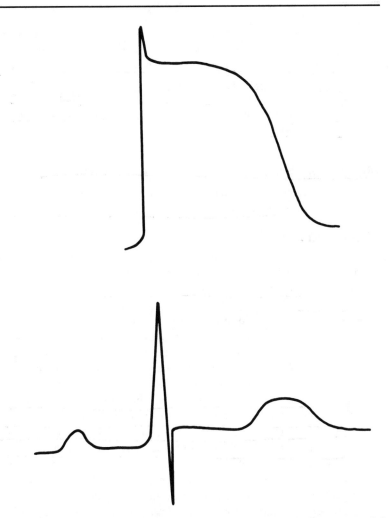

Figure 1.5. Relationship between the ventricular action potential (top) and the surface ECG (bottom). The rapid depolarization phase (phase 0) is reflected by the QRS complex on the ECG. Because phase 0 is almost instantaneous, the QRS complex yields directional information on ventricular depolarization. In contrast, the repolarization portion of the action potential (phases 1–3) has significant duration. Consequently, the portion of the surface ECG that reflects repolarization (the ST segment and the T wave) yields little directional information.

mation, and abnormalities in the ST segments and T waves are most often (and quite properly) interpreted as being nonspecific. The QT interval represents the time from the beginning of depolarization (the beginning of the QRS complex) to the end of repolarization (the end of the T wave) of the ventricular myocardium, and thus reflects the average action potential duration of ventricular muscle.

MECHANISMS OF CARDIAC TACHYARRHYTHMIAS

Rapid cardiac arrhythmias are generally caused by one of three mechanisms: abnormal automaticity, reentry, or triggered activity.

Automaticity

As already noted, automaticity is an important feature of the normal electrical system; the pacemaker function of the heart depends on it. Under some circumstances, however, abnormal automaticity can occur. When an abnormal acceleration of phase 4 activity occurs at some location within the heart, an automatic tachyarrhythmia is the result. Such an automatic focus can arise in the atria, the AV junction, or the ventricles and can lead to automatic atrial tachycardia, automatic junctional tachycardia, or automatic ventricular tachycardia.

Automatic tachyarrhythmias are not particularly common; they probably account for less than 10% of all tachyarrhythmias. Further, automatic tachyarrhythmias are usually recognizable by their characteristics and the clinical settings in which they occur.

Consideration of some of the features of sinus tachycardia, which is a *normal* automatic tachycardia, may be helpful in this regard. Sinus tachycardia usually occurs as a result of appropriately increased sympathetic tone (e.g., in response to exercise). When sinus tachycardia develops, the heart rate gradually increases from the basic (resting) sinus rate; when sinus tachycardia subsides, the rate likewise decreases gradually.

Similarly, automatic tachyarrhythmias often display "warmup" and "warm-down" in rate when the arrhythmia begins and ends. Also analogous to sinus tachycardia, automatic tachyarrhythmias often have metabolic causes, such as acute cardiac ischemia, hypoxemia, hypokalemia, hypomagnesemia, acid–base disturbances, high sympathetic tone, or the use of sympathomimetic agents. Therefore, automatic arrhythmias are frequently seen in acutely ill patients, usually in the intensive care unit (ICU) setting.

Common examples of automatic tachyarrhythmias are the multifocal atrial tachycardias that accompany acute exacerbations of chronic pulmonary disease, many of the atrial and ventricular tachyarrhythmias seen during the induction of and recovery from general anesthesia (probably a result of surges in sympathetic tone), and the ventricular arrhythmias seen during the first minutes to hours of an acute myocardial infarction (enhanced automaticity in this situation is thought to be mediated by ischemia).

Of all tachyarrhythmias, automatic arrhythmias are closest to resembling an "itch" of the heart. The balm of antiarrhythmic drugs is occasionally helpful, but the primary treatment of these arrhythmias should always be directed toward identifying and treating the underlying metabolic cause. In general, the ICU arrhythmias resolve once the patient's acute medical problems have been stabilized.

Reentry

The mechanism of reentry accounts for most clinically significant tachyarrhythmias. Recognition of this fact and of the fact that reentrant arrhythmias are amenable to study in the laboratory led to widespread proliferation of electrophysiology laboratories during the past 2 decades.

The mechanism of reentry, although less intuitive than the mechanism of automaticity, can still be reduced to a few simple concepts. Reentry requires meeting certain criteria (Figure 1.6). First, two roughly parallel conducting pathways must be connected proximally and distally by conducting tissue, which forms a potential electrical circuit. Second, one pathway must have a longer refractory period than the other pathway. Third, the pathway with the shorter refractory period must conduct electrical impulses more slowly than does the opposite pathway.

If all these seemingly implausible conditions are met, reentry can be initiated by introducing an appropriately timed premature impulse to the circuit (Figure 1.7). The premature impulse must enter the circuit precisely at a time when the pathway with the long refractory period is still refractory from the latest depolarization and at a time when the pathway with the shorter refractory period has recovered and is able to conduct the premature impulse. The impulse enters the pathway with the shorter refractory period but is conducted slowly because that pathway has the electrophysiologic property of slow conduction. By the time the impulse reaches the long-refractory-period pathway from below,

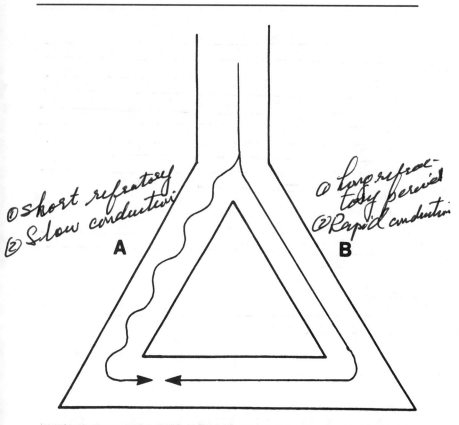

Figure 1.6. Prerequisites for reentry. An anatomic circuit must be present in which two portions of the circuit (pathways A and B) have electrophysiologic properties that differ from one another in a critical way. In this example, pathway A conducts electrical impulses more slowly than pathway B; pathway B has a longer refractory period than pathway A.

that pathway has had time to recover and is able to conduct the impulse in the retrograde direction. If the retrograde impulse now reenters the first pathway and is conducted antegradely (as is likely because of the short refractory period of the first pathway), a continuously circulating impulse is established, which rotates around and around the reentrant circuit. All that is necessary for the reentrant impulse to usurp the rhythm of the heart is for the impulse to exit from the circuit at some point during each lap and thereby depolarize the remaining myocardium outside the circuit.

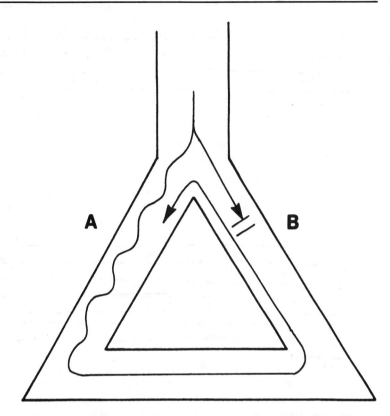

Figure 1.7. Initiation of reentry. If the prerequisites described in Figure 1.6 are present, an appropriately timed premature electrical impulse can block in pathway B (which has a relatively long refractory period) while conducting down pathway A. Because conduction down pathway A is slow, pathway B has time to recover, allowing the impulse to conduct retrogradely up pathway B. The impulse can then reenter pathway A. A continuously circulating impulse is thus established.

Because reentry depends on critical differences in the conduction velocities and refractory periods among the various pathways of the circuit and because conduction velocities and refractory periods, as we have seen, are determined by the shape of the action potential, the action potentials of the two pathways are different from one another. Thus drugs that change the shape of the action potential might be useful in the treatment of reentrant arrhythmias.

Reentrant circuits occur with some frequency in the human heart. Some reentrant circuits are present at birth, notably those causing supraventricular tachycardias (e.g., reentry associated with AV bypass tracts and with dual AV nodal tracts). However, reentrant circuits that cause ventricular tachycardias are almost never congenital, but come into existence as cardiac disease develops during life. In the ventricles, reentrant circuits arise in areas in which normal cardiac tissue becomes interspersed with patches of fibrous (scar) tissue, thus forming potential anatomic circuits. Thus, ventricular reentrant circuits usually occur only when fibrosis develops in the ventricles, such as after a myocardial infarction or with cardiomyopathic diseases.

Theoretically, if all anatomic and electrophysiologic criteria for reentry are present, any impulse that enters the circuit at the appropriate instant in time induces a reentrant tachycardia. The time from the end of the refractory period of the shorter-refractory-period pathway to the end of the refractory period of the pathway with a longer refractory time, during which reentry can be induced, is called the *tachycardia zone*. Treating reentrant arrhythmias often involves trying to narrow or abolish the tachycardia zone (by increasing the refractory period of the shorter-time pathway or decreasing the refractory period of the longer-time pathway).

Because reentrant arrhythmias can be reproducibly induced (and terminated) by appropriately timed impulses, these arrhythmias are ideal for study in the electrophysiology laboratory. In many instances (very commonly with supraventricular arrhythmias, but only occasionally with ventricular arrhythmias), the pathways involved in the reentrant circuit can be precisely mapped, the effect of various therapies can be assessed, and critical portions of the circuit can even be ablated through the electrode catheter.

Triggered Activity

Triggered activity is a third mechanism of tachyarrhythmias that has some features of both automaticity and reentry. Like automaticity, triggered activity involves the movement of positive ions into the cardiac cell. Rather than causing the sort of gradual positive deflection one sees during phase 4 automaticity, however, in triggered activity, the ionic fluxes cause a rather acute "bump" (Figure 1.8) during late phase 3 or early phase 4. The bump is called an *afterdepolarization*. If afterdepolarizations are large enough, they can engage the rapid sodium channels (which, as noted, are voltage dependent), and thus generate another action potential (see Figure 1.8). Therefore, triggered activity resembles automaticity in that

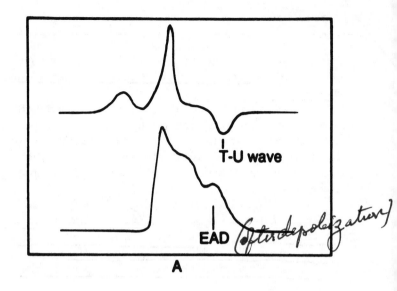

T-U wave

EAD *(afterdepolarization)*

A

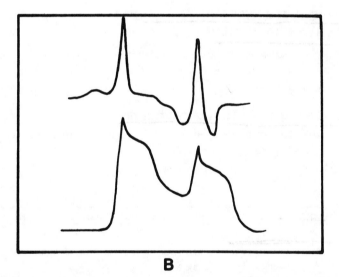

B

Figure 1.8. Triggered activity. Both panels show a surface ECG (top) and a simultaneous ventricular action potential (bottom). A. Phase 3 of the action potential is interrupted by a "bump"—an EAD. The EAD is reflected on the surface ECG by a prolonged and distorted T wave (T-U wave). B. The EAD is of sufficient amplitude to engage the rapid sodium channel and generate another action potential. The resultant premature complex is seen on surface ECG. Note that just as the premature action potential is coincident with the EAD (since it is generated by the EAD), the premature ventricular complex is also coincident with the T-U wave of the previous complex.

new action potentials can be generated by leakage of positive ions into the cell. Many experts classify triggered activity as a subset of automaticity.

However, unlike automaticity (and like reentry), triggered activity is not always spontaneous (and therefore not truly automatic). Triggered activity, like reentry, can sometimes be provoked by appropriately timed premature beats. Thus, like reentry, triggered activity can sometimes be induced with programmed pacing techniques.

The clinical significance of triggered activity has become clearer during the past few years. Digitalis-toxic arrhythmias, torsades de pointes, and the rare cases of ventricular tachycardia that respond to calcium-blocking agents have all been advanced as arrhythmias that are most likely caused by triggered activity.

CLINICAL FEATURES OF THE MAJOR TACHYARRHYTHMIAS

Before considering how antiarrhythmic drugs work, it is helpful to review the salient clinical features of the major cardiac tachyarrhythmias.

Supraventricular Tachyarrhythmias

Table 1.1 classifies the supraventricular tachyarrhythmias according to mechanism.

Table 1.1. Classification of Supraventricular Tachyarrhythmias

Automatic arrhythmias
    Some atrial tachycardias associated with acute medical conditions
    Some mulitfocal atrial tachycardias
Reentrant arrhythmias
    SA nodal reentrant tachycardia
    Intra-atrial reentrant tachycardia
    Atrial flutter and atrial fibrillation
    AV nodal reentrant tachycardia
    Macroreentrant (bypass-mediated) reentrant tachycardia
Triggered arrhythmias (probable mechanism)
    Digitalis-toxic atrial tachycardia
    Some multifocal atrial tachycardias

SA = sinoatrial; AV = atrioventricular.

Automatic Supraventricular Tachyarrhythmias: Automatic supraventricular arrhythmias are seen almost exclusively in acutely ill patients, most of whom have one of the following conditions: myocardial ischemia, acute exacerbations of chronic lung disease, acute alcohol toxicity, or major electrolyte disturbances. Any of these disorders can produce ectopic automatic foci in the atrial myocardium.

Clinically, the rate of automatic atrial tachycardias is usually less than 200 beats/min. Like all automatic rhythms, the onset and offset are usually relatively gradual, that is, often display warm up, in which the heart rate accelerates (or decelerates) over several cycles. Each QRS complex is preceded by a discrete P wave, whose shape generally differs from the normal sinus P wave, depending on the location of the automatic focus within the atrium. Likewise, the PR interval is often shorter than it is during sinus rhythm since the ectopic focus may be relatively close to the AV node. Because automatic atrial tachycardias arise in and are localized to the atrial myocardium (and thus the arrhythmia itself is not dependent on the AV node), if AV block is produced, atrial arrhythmia itself is unaffected.

Multifocal atrial tachycardia (Figure 1.9) is the most common form of automatic atrial tachycardia. It is characterized by multiple (usually at least three) P wave morphologies, and irregular PP intervals. Multifocal atrial tachycardia is thought to be caused by the presence of several automatic foci within the atria, firing at different rates. The arrhythmia is usually associated with exacerbation of chronic lung disease, especially in patients receiving theophylline.

Pharmacologic therapy is usually not very helpful in treating automatic atrial tachycardia, though drugs that affect the AV node can slow the ventricular rate by creating second-degree block. The basic strategy for treating automatic atrial arrhythmias is to aggressively treat the underlying illness.

Reentrant Supraventricular Tachyarrhythmias: In general, patients have reentrant supraventricular tachyarrhythmias because they are born with abnormal electrical pathways that create potential reentrant circuits. Accordingly (in contrast to patients with automatic supraventricular arrhythmias), these patients most often initially experience symptoms when they are young and healthy. Most supraventricular tachyarrhythmias seen in otherwise healthy patients are caused by the mechanism of reentry.

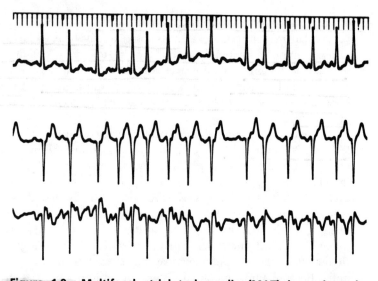

Figure 1.9. Multifocal atrial tachycardia (MAT) is an irregular atrial tachyarrhythmia that superficially resembles atrial fibrillation. However, in MAT (in contrast to atrial fibrillation) each QRS complex is preceded by a discrete P wave. Further, at least three distinct P wave morphologies are present, which reflects the multifocal origin of atrial activity in this arrhythmia.

The five general categories of reentrant supraventricular arrhythmias are listed in Table 1.1. Many clinicians lump these arrhythmias together (except for atrial fibrillation and flutter, which generally are easily distinguishable), as paroxysmal atrial tachycardia (PAT). In most instances, however, an astute clinician can tell which specific category of arrhythmia he or she is dealing with (and therefore can institute appropriate therapy) merely by carefully examining a 12-lead ECG of the arrhythmia.

AV Nodal Reentrant Tachycardia: AV nodal reentrant tachycardia is the most common type of PAT and accounts for nearly 60% of regular supraventricular tachyarrhythmias. In AV nodal reentry, the reentrant circuit can be visualized as being enclosed entirely within an AV node that is functionally divided into two separate pathways (Figure 1.10). The dual pathways form the reentrant circuit responsible for the arrhythmia. Because the reentrant circuit is within the AV node, the pharmacologic treatment of AV nodal reentry usually involves giving drugs whose major site of action is the AV node.

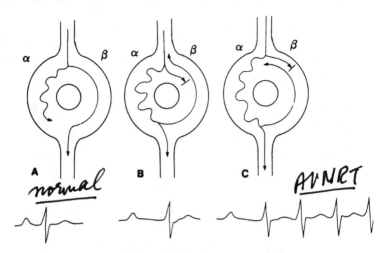

Figure 1.10. AV nodal reentrant tachycardia. A. In patients with AV nodal reentry, the AV node is functionally divided into two separate pathways (alpha (α) and beta (β) pathways). Similar to the example shown in Figures 1.6 and 1.7, the alpha pathway conducts more slowly than the beta pathway, and the beta pathway has a longer refractory period than that of the alpha pathway. Since the beta pathway conducts more rapidly than does the alpha pathway, a normal atrial impulse reaches the ventricles via the beta pathway. B. A premature atrial impulse can find the beta pathway still refractory at a time when the alpha pathway is not refractory. Because conduction down the alpha pathway is slow, the resultant PR interval is prolonged. C. If conditions are right, a premature impulse can block in the beta pathway and conduct down the alpha pathway (as in B), then travel retrograde up the beta pathway and reenter the alpha pathway in the antegrade direction. AV nodal reentrant tachycardia results when such a circuitous impulse is established within the AV node.

Bypass-Tract-Mediated Macroreentrant Tachycardia: Tachycardia mediated by AV bypass tracts is the next most common type of reentrant supraventricular tachycardia and accounts for approximately 30% of arrhythmias presenting as PAT. Most patients with such bypass tracts do not have overt Wolff-Parkinson-White syndrome, however. Instead, they have *concealed* bypass tracts, that is, bypass tracts that are incapable of conducting in the antegrade direction (from the atrium to the ventricles) and therefore never display delta waves. Concealed bypass tracts are able to conduct electrical impulses only in the retrograde direction (from the ventricles to the atrium).

The reentrant circuit responsible for these tachycardias is formed by the bypass tract, which almost always constitutes the retrograde pathway, and the normal AV nodal conducting system (the antegrade pathway) connected by the atrial and ventricular myocardium (Figure 1.11). Because the reentrant circuit is large (involving the AV node, the His–Purkinje system, the ventricular myocardium, the bypass tract, and the atrial myocardium), it is termed a *macroreentrant circuit*. Also, because the circuit consists of

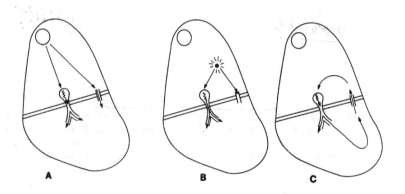

Figure 1.11. Bypass-tract-mediated macroreentrant tachycardia.
(A) Because a bypass tract is present, a normal sinus beat is transmitted to the ventricles via two separate pathways. Because the ventricle is partially preexcited (i.e., some ventricular myocardium is depolarized early via the bypass tract), the QRS complex displays a delta wave. A bypass tract usually has a longer refractory period than the normal conducting system, and the normal conducting system includes the slow-conducting AV node and conducts electrical impulses more slowly than the bypass tract. Thus, the substrate for reentry is present. **(B)** A premature atrial complex (PAC) occurs during the refractory period of the bypass tract and is therefore conducted solely via the normal conducting system. The resultant QRS complex displays no delta wave. **(C)** Because conduction via the normal conducting system is relatively slow, the bypass tract may no longer be refractory by the time the impulse reaches the ventricles. Thus, the bypass tract may be able to conduct the impulse retrogradely back to the atrium. If so, a reentrant impulse may be established, which travels antegradely down the normal conducting system and retrogradely up the bypass tract. The result is a large (macro) reentrant circuit.

several types of tissue, it can be attacked on many levels by many different kinds of drugs—drugs that affect the AV node, the bypass tract, the ventricular myocardium, or the atrial myocardium.

Intra-atrial Reentry: Intra-atrial reentry accounts for only a small percentage of arrhythmias presenting as PAT. The reentrant circuit in intra-atrial reentry resides entirely within the atrial myocardium and does not involve the AV conducting system (Figure 1.12). Intra-atrial reentry resembles automatic atrial tachycardia because discrete (often bizarre) P waves precede each QRS complex, and AV block can occur without affecting the arrhythmia itself. Intra-atrial reentry differs from automatic tachycardia because of its sudden onset and termination, and, like all reentrant arrhythmias, it can be induced by pacing. Intra-atrial reentry is affected only by drugs that affect the atrial myocardium.

Atrial Flutter and Atrial Fibrillation: Atrial flutter and fibrillation are special forms of intra-atrial reentrant tachycardias and are

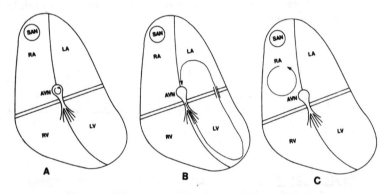

Figure 1.12. The components of the reentrant circuit determine which antiarrhythmic drugs are likely to be effective in treating supraventricular tachycardia. Both AV nodal reentry (A) and macroreentry (B) include the AV node within the reentrant circuit. Therefore, drugs that affect the AV node affect the reentrant circuit itself and may be useful in terminating or preventing the arrhythmia. In contrast, in intra-atrial reentry (C) the reentrant circuit does not include the AV node. Drugs that affect the AV node generally do not affect intra-atrial reentry itself, although they may be effective in slowing the ventricular response during the arrhythmia. Atrial fibrillation, atrial flutter, and automatic atrial tachycardia are similar to intra-atrial reentry in that the AV node is not required for initiating or sustaining these arrhythmias. AVN = atrioventricular node; LA = left atrium; LV = left ventricle; RA = right atrium; RV = right ventricle; SAN = sinoatrial node.

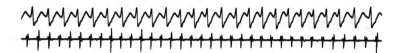

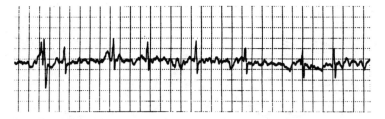

Figure 1.13. Atrial flutter. A surface ECG (top) and an intracardiac electrogram that directly records intra-atrial electrical activity (bottom) are shown. Note the two atrial impulses (seen on the intracardiac electrogram) for every QRS complex; AV block occurs in a typical 2:1 pattern. Only a hint of the classic sawtooth pattern shows on the surface ECG in this tracing. This is also a typical finding—often, a higher degree of block must be provoked (e.g., with carotid sinus massage) for the diagnosis of atrial flutter to become clear.

Figure 1.14. Atrial fibrillation. Note the randomly irregular ventricular response and the absence of discrete P waves.

generally distinguishable from other kinds of atrial tachyarrhythmias (commonly labeled PAT) by reviewing a 12-lead ECG.

In atrial flutter, the atrial activity is regular, in excess of 220 beats/min, and usually displays a typical sawtooth pattern (Figure 1.13). Atrial flutter is almost always accompanied by AV block, most often in a 2:1 pattern.

In atrial fibrillation, the atrial activity is continuous and chaotic, and discrete P waves cannot be distinguished (Figure 1.14). The ventricular response is completely irregular, which reflects the chaotic nature of the atrial activity.

Since atrial fibrillation and flutter are intra-atrial arrhythmias, AV block (which occurs in almost every case) does not affect the arrhythmia itself. Drug therapy is usually aimed at converting the arrhythmia by use of drugs that affect the atrial myocardium or controlling the ventricular response with drugs that affect AV conduction.

SA Nodal Reentry: SA nodal reentry is a relatively uncommon arrhythmia in which the reentrant circuit is thought to be enclosed entirely within the SA node (i.e., dual SA nodal pathways are thought to exist, similar to those seen in AV nodal reentry). Discrete P waves identical to sinus P waves precede each QRS complex. SA nodal reentry is distinguishable from normal sinus tachycardia (which is automatic in mechanism) by its sudden onset and offset and by its inducibility with pacing. It is affected by drugs that affect the SA and AV nodes.

Triggered Supraventricular Tachyarrhythmias: The only supraventricular tachycardia commonly attributed to triggered activity is that seen with digitalis toxicity. Digitalis toxicity can produce delayed afterdepolarizations (DADs) that can lead to atrial tachycardias. Clinically, since digitalis also produces AV block, digitalis toxic arrhythmia often presents as atrial tachycardia with block. In fact, the presence of atrial tachycardia with block should always make one consider the possibility of digitalis toxicity.

Electrocardiographic Patterns of Supraventricular Tachyarrhythmias: Often one can specifically diagnose a patient's supraventricular arrhythmia by examining a 12-lead ECG. Atrial flutter and atrial fibrillation can usually be distinguished by simple inspection. In the supraventricular tachycardias commonly labeled PAT (regular, narrow-complex tachycardias), both the relationship of the P waves to the QRS complexes and the morphology of the P waves during the tachycardia can be very helpful. Figure 1.15 shows the essential electrocardiographic characteristics of the four types of reentry that are commonly grouped under the heading PAT.

Ventricular Tachyarrhythmias

Table 1.2 classifies the ventricular tachyarrhythmias according to mechanism.

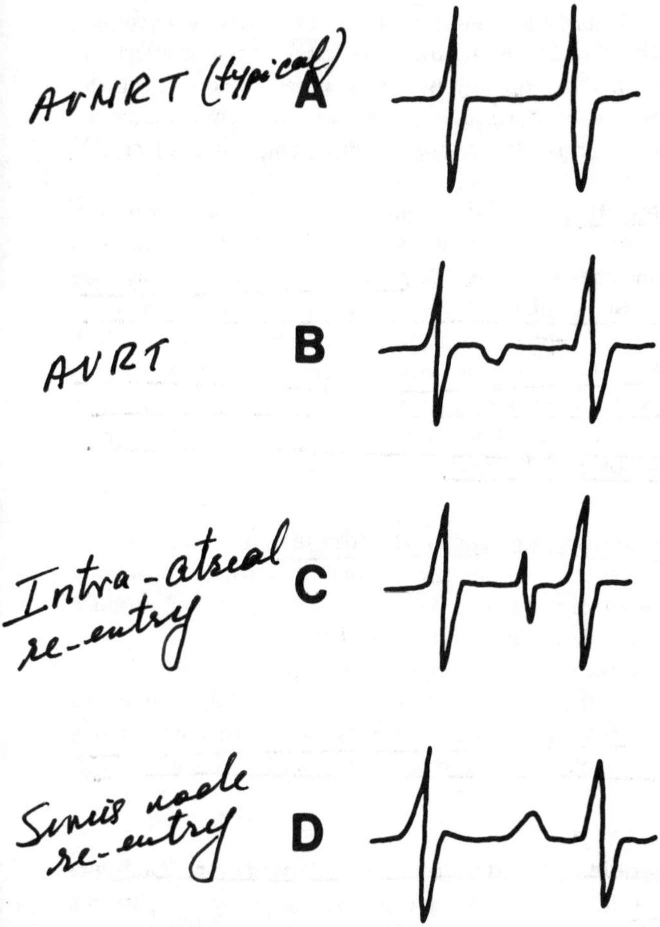

AVNRT (typical) **A**

AVRT **B**

Intra-atrial re-entry **C**

Sinus node re-entry **D**

Figure 1.15. Typical P wave relationships in four kinds of PAT. Surface ECG lead II is depicted. (A) In AV nodal reentrant tachycardia, the P wave is usually buried within the QRS complex and is most often not discernible even with careful study of all 12 ECG leads. (B) In bypass-tract-mediated macroreentrant tachycardia, the inferior ECG leads usually show a negative P wave (it has a superior axis because the atria are activated in the retrograde direction). Also, the P wave is usually closer to the preceding QRS complex than to the following QRS complex. (C) In intra-atrial reentry, discrete P waves almost always are seen before each QRS complex. Because the intra-atrial reentrant circuit can be located anywhere within the atria, the P wave morphology can have any configuration. The PR interval is usually normal or short. (D) In SA nodal reentry, P waves and the PR interval appear normal.

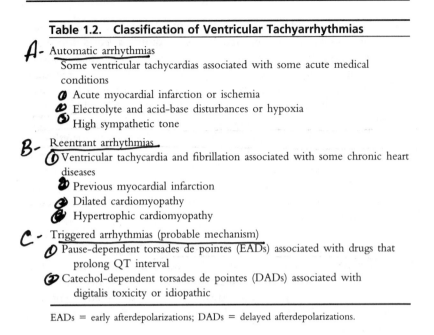

Table 1.2. Classification of Ventricular Tachyarrhythmias

A - Automatic arrhythmias

Some ventricular tachycardias associated with some acute medical conditions

ⓐ Acute myocardial infarction or ischemia

ⓑ Electrolyte and acid-base disturbances or hypoxia

ⓒ High sympathetic tone

B - Reentrant arrhythmias

ⓓ Ventricular tachycardia and fibrillation associated with some chronic heart diseases

ⓔ Previous myocardial infarction

ⓕ Dilated cardiomyopathy

ⓖ Hypertrophic cardiomyopathy

C - Triggered arrhythmias (probable mechanism)

ⓗ Pause-dependent torsades de pointes (EADs) associated with drugs that prolong QT interval

ⓘ Catechol-dependent torsades de pointes (DADs) associated with digitalis toxicity or idiopathic

EADs = early afterdepolarizations; DADs = delayed afterdepolarizations.

Automatic Ventricular Tachyarrhythmias: Abnormal automaticity accounts for a relatively small proportion of ventricular tachyarrhythmias. As in automatic atrial arrhythmias, automatic ventricular arrhythmias are usually associated with acute medical conditions such as myocardial ischemia, acid–base disturbances, electrolyte abnormalities, and high adrenergic tone. Patients with automatic ventricular arrhythmias most often are having acute myocardial ischemia or infarction or are suffering from some other acute medical illness. Most arrhythmias occurring within the first few hours of an acute myocardial infarction are thought to be automatic. Once the ischemic tissue dies or stabilizes, the substrate for automaticity is no longer present.

In general, treatment of automatic ventricular arrhythmias consists of treating the underlying illness. Antiarrhythmic drugs are occasionally beneficial.

Reentrant Ventricular Tachyarrhythmias: Most ventricular arrhythmias are reentrant in mechanism. Although the conditions producing automatic ventricular arrhythmias are usually temporary (e.g., cardiac ischemia), the substrate necessary for reentrant ventricular arrhythmias, once present, tends to be permanent.

Reentrant circuits within the ventricles usually arise after scar tissue forms in the ventricular myocardium, a condition most commonly seen in patients who have myocardial infarctions or cardiomyopathy. Once the scar tissue gives rise to a reentrant circuit, the circuit is always present, and the potential for a ventricular arrhythmia always exists. Thus, the "late" sudden deaths that occur after a myocardial infarction (from 12 hr to several years after the acute event) are usually a result of reentrant arrhythmias. Reentrant ventricular arrhythmias are seen only rarely in individuals who have normal ventricles.

Most antiarrhythmic drugs affect the ventricular myocardium and, accordingly, most are used to treat ventricular tachyarrhythmias.

Triggered Ventricular Tachyarrhythmias: Triggered activity is a relatively uncommon cause of ventricular arrhythmias but is seen often enough that one must be alert to its existence, especially since the etiologies and treatments of triggered ventricular arrhythmias are very different from the more common arrhythmias.

Two fairly distinct clinical syndromes have been identified involving triggered activity: catechol-dependent arrhythmias and pause-dependent arrhythmias. In each syndrome, the arrhythmias tend to be polymorphic and have been referred to as *torsades de pointes.*

Catechol-Dependent Triggered Arrhythmias: Catechol-dependent triggered arrhythmias are caused by DADs that occur during phase 4 of the action potential (Figure 1.16A). DADs occur in the setting of digitalis intoxication, cardiac ischemia, and in certain patients who have a congenital form of QT prolongation. The latter patients have been postulated to have an imbalance in the sympathetic innervation of the heart, with predominant input coming from the left stellate ganglia—stimulation of which can reproduce DADs.

The arrhythmias typically are polymorphic and are seen in conditions of high sympathetic tone. Patients with catechol-dependent triggered activity therefore experience arrhythmias (often manifested by syncope or cardiac arrest) in times of severe emotional stress or during exercise. Often they have normal ECGs at rest but develop QT abnormalities during exercise. The onset of the arrhythmia is not associated with a pause.

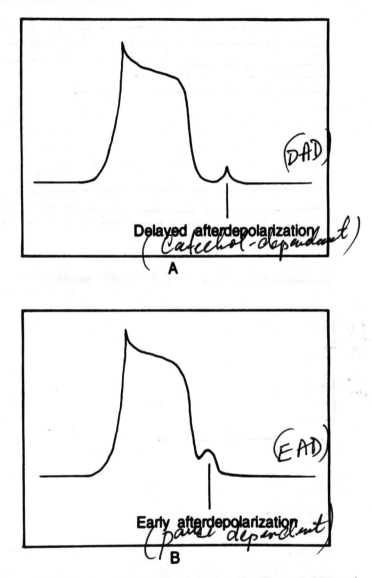

Figure 1.16. Early and delayed afterdepolarizations. A. DADs of the type thought to be responsible for catechol-dependent triggered arrhythmias. The DAD occurs after the end of phase 3. B. EAD of the type thought to be responsible for pause-dependent triggered arrhythmias. The EAD occurs during phase 3.

Left stellate sympathectomy has eliminated arrhythmias in some patients. Medical treatment has generally consisted of beta blockers and calcium-channel blockers (because DADs are thought to be mediated by calcium channels).

Pause-Dependent Triggered Arrhythmias: Pause-dependent triggered arrhythmias are caused by afterdepolarizations that occur during phase 3 of the action potential; hence, they are called *early afterdepolarizations* (EADs) (see Figure 1.16B). If the EAD reaches the threshold potential of the cardiac cell, another action potential can be generated, and an arrhythmia occurs. EADs are generally seen only under circumstances that prolong the duration of the action potential, such as electrolyte abnormalities (hypokalemia and hypomagnesemia), and with the use of drugs, predominantly antiarrhythmic drugs (Table 1.3).

Table 1.3. Drugs that Can Cause Torsades de Pointes

Class I and Class III antiarrhythmic drugs

1A — Quinidine
— Procainamide
— Disopyramide
1C — Propafenone
III — Sotalol
— Amiodarone
— Bretylium
— Ibutilide

Tricyclic and tetracyclic antidepressants
    Amitriptyline
    Imipramine
    Doxepin
    Maprotiline

Phenothiazines
    Thioridazine
    Chlorpromazine

Antibiotics
    Erythromycin
    Trimethoprim-Sulfamethoxazole

Others
    Bepridil
    Lidoflazine
    Probucol
    Haloperidol
    Chloral hydrate

Most likely, some finite subset of the normal population is susceptible to developing EADs. Susceptible individuals probably have an inborn subclinical abnormality of the cardiac cell membrane that becomes manifest only when action potential duration is increased by drugs or electrolyte abnormalities.

The resulting arrhythmias are typically polymorphic and tend to occur repeatedly and in short bursts, although prolonged epi-

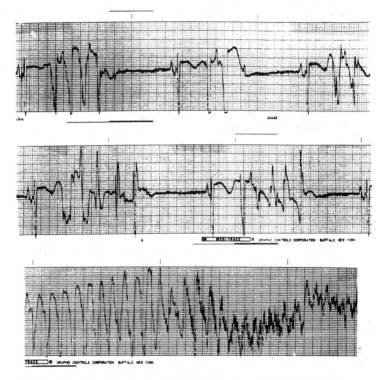

Figure 1.17. Pause-dependent triggered arrhythmias. The figure depicts rhythm strips from a patient who developed torsades de pointes after receiving a Class IA antiarrhythmic agent. The top two strips show the typical pattern—each burst of polymorphic ventricular tachycardia is followed by a compensatory pause; the pause, in turn, causes the ensuing sinus beat to be followed by another burst of ventricular tachycardia. The bottom strip shows the sustained polymorphic ventricular tachycardia that followed after several minutes of ventricular tachycardia bigeminy. Note the broad T-U wave that follows each sinus beat in the top two strips. The T-U wave is thought to reflect the pause-dependent EADs that are probably responsible for the arrhythmia.

sodes leading to death can occur. The repolarization abnormalities responsible for these arrhythmias (i.e., the afterdepolarizations) are reflected on the surface ECG—the T wave configuration is often distorted, and a U wave is present. The U wave is probably the surface manifestation of the EAD itself. The T-U abnormalities tend to be dynamic; that is, they wax and wane mainly depending on heart rate. The slower the heart rate, the more exaggerated the T-U abnormality; hence, this condition is said to be pause dependent. Once a burst of ventricular tachycardia is generated (triggered by an EAD that is so exaggerated that it reaches threshold potential), it tends to be repeated in a pattern of ventricular tachycardia bigeminy. An example is shown in Figure 1.17. In this figure, each

Table 1.4. Clinical Features of Uncommon Ventricular Tachycardias

① Idiopathic left ventricular tachycardia
  Younger patients, no structural heart disease
  Inducible VT with RBBB, superior axis morphology
  Responds to beta blockers and calcium-channel blockers
  Both reentry and triggered activity have been postulated as mechanisms

② Right ventricular outflow tract tachycardia (repetitive monomorphic VT)
  Younger patients, no structural heart disease
  VT originates in RV outflow tract; has LBBB, inferior axis morphology; often not inducible during EP testing
  Responds to beta blockers, calcium blockers, and transcatheter RF ablation
  Postulated to be due to automaticity or triggered automaticity

③ Ventricular tachycardia associated with right ventricular dysplasia
  fatty Younger patients with RV dysplasia (portions of RV replaced by fibrous tissue) CT, MRI Rx: ICD
  LBBB ventricular tachycardia; almost always inducible during EP testing
  Treatment similar to treatment of reentrant VT in setting of coronary artery disease

④ Bundle branch reentry
  Patients with dilated cardiomyopathy and intraventricular conduction abnormality
  Rapid VT with LBBB morphology; reentrant circuit uses RBB in downward direction and LBB in upward direction
  Can be cured by RF ablation of RBB

EP = electrophysiologic; LBB = left bundle branch; LBBB = left bundle branch block; RBB = right bundle branch; RBBB = right bundle branch block; RV = right ventricle; VT = ventricular tachycardia.

burst of polymorphic ventricular tachycardia causes a compensatory pause, and the pause causes the ensuing sinus beat to be associated with pronounced U wave abnormalities (i.e., a large EAD is generated). The large EAD, in turn, produces another burst of tachycardia. Pause-dependent triggered activity should be strongly suspected whenever this ECG pattern is seen—especially in the setting of overt QT prolongation or in the setting of conditions that predispose to QT prolongation.

The acute treatment of pause-dependent triggered activity consists of attempting to reduce the duration of the action potential, to eliminate the pauses, or both. Drugs that prolong the QT interval should be immediately discontinued and avoided. Electrolyte abnormalities should be corrected quickly. Intravenous magnesium often ameliorates the arrhythmias even when serum magnesium levels are in the normal range. The mainstay of emergent treatment of the arrhythmias, however, is to eliminate the pauses that trigger the arrhythmias by increasing the heart rate. This is most often accomplished by pacing the atrium or the ventricles (usually, at rates of 100 to 120 beats/min) or, occasionally, by using an isoproterenol infusion.

Once the underlying cause for the EADs has been reversed, chronic treatment focuses on avoiding conditions that prolong action potential duration.

Miscellaneous Ventricular Arrhythmias: Several clinical syndromes have been described involving unusual ventricular arrhythmias that do not fit clearly into any category. Nomenclature for these arrhythmias is unsettled in the literature, which reflects the lack of understanding of these arrhythmias. Table 1.4 lists the salient features of relatively uncommon ventricular arrhythmias.

Introduction to Antiarrhythmic Drugs

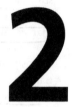

All cardiac tachyarrhythmias—whether caused by abnormal automaticity, reentry, or triggered activity—are mediated by localized or generalized changes in the cardiac action potential. Thus, it should not be surprising that drugs that alter the action potential might have important effects on cardiac arrhythmias. This chapter considers how antiarrhythmic drugs work and how they are classified.

HOW ANTIARRHYTHMIC DRUGS WORK

Thinking of an antiarrhythmic drug as a soothing balm that suppresses the irritation of cardiac arrhythmias is more than merely naive; it is dangerous. If this is how one imagines antiarrhythmic drugs, when an arrhythmia fails to respond to a chosen drug, the natural response is either to increase the dosage of the drug, or worse, to add additional drugs (in a futile attempt to sufficiently sooth the irritation).

Effect on Cardiac Action Potential

What antiarrhythmic drugs actually do—the characteristic that makes them "antiarrhythmic"—is change the shape of the cardiac action potential. Antiarrhythmic drugs do this, in general, by altering the channels that control the flow of ions across the cardiac cell membrane.

Class I antiarrhythmic drugs inhibit the rapid sodium channel. As shown in Figure 2.1, the rapid sodium channel is controlled by the m gate and the h gate. In the resting state, the m gate is open *closed* and the h gate is closed. *open* When an appropriate stimulus occurs, the

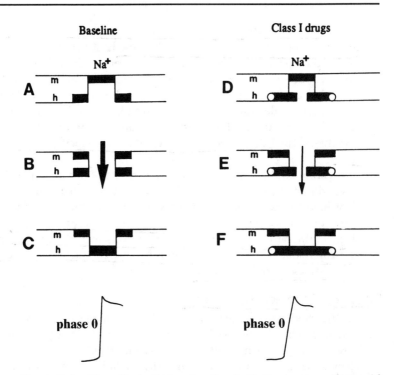

Figure 2.1. The effect of Class I antiarrhythmic drugs on the rapid sodium channel. The sodium channel (Na^+) is controlled by two gates: the m gate and the h gate. Panels A through C display the function of the two controlling gates in the baseline (drug-free) state. A The resting state; the m gate is closed and the h gate is open. B The cell is stimulated, causing the m gate to open, which allows positively charged sodium ions to rapidly enter the cell (large arrow). C The h gate shuts and sodium transport stops (i.e., phase 0 ends). Panels D through E display the effect of adding a Class I antiarrhythmic drug (open circles). D Class I drug binding to the h gate, which makes the h gate behave as if it is partially closed. E. The cell is stimulated; the m gate still opens normally, but the channel through which sodium ions enter the cell is narrower, and sodium transport is slower. Consequently, reaching the end of phase 0 takes longer; the slope of Phase 0 and the conduction velocity are decreased.

m gate opens, which allows positively charged sodium ions to pour into the cell and causes the cell to depolarize (phase 0 of the action potential). After a few milliseconds, the h gate closes and sodium stops flowing; phase 0 ends.

Class I antiarrhythmic drugs work by binding to the h gate, making it behave as if it is partially closed. When the m gate opens, the opening through which sodium enters the cell is functionally much narrower; thus, it takes longer to depolarize the cell (i.e., the slope of phase 0 is decreased). Because the speed of depolarization determines how quickly adjacent cells depolarize (and therefore affects the speed of conduction of the electrical impulse), Class I drugs decrease the conduction velocity of cardiac tissue.

Although the precise sites of action have not been completely worked out, most other antiarrhythmic drugs operate similarly; they bind to the channels and gates that control the flux of ions across the cardiac cell membrane. In so doing, the drugs change the shape of the cardiac action potential and thus change the three basic electrophysiologic properties of cardiac tissue: conduction velocity, refractoriness, and automaticity.

Effect on Cardiac Arrhythmias

Tachyarrhythmias are mediated by changes in the cardiac action potential, whether the mechanism is automaticity, reentry, or triggered activity. It is not difficult to imagine, then, how drugs that change the shape of the action potential might be useful in treating cardiac tachyarrhythmias.

In practice, the drugs commonly referred to as antiarrhythmic are relatively ineffective in treating automatic or triggered arrhythmias. Instead, the potential benefit of these drugs is almost exclusive to the treatment of reentrant arrhythmias, which account for most cardiac arrhythmias. Nonetheless, drugs that change the shape of the action potential can potentially affect all three mechanisms of arrhythmias.

Automatic Arrhythmias: Abnormal automaticity, whether atrial or ventricular, is generally seen in patients who are acutely ill and as a result have significant metabolic abnormalities. The metabolic abnormalities appear to change the characteristics of phase 4 of the cardiac action potential. The changes that most likely account for enhanced abnormal automaticity are an increased slope of phase 4 depolarization or a reduced maximum diastolic potential (i.e., a reduced negativity in the transmembrane potential at the beginning of phase 4). Either change can cause the rapid, spontaneous generation of action potentials and thus precipitate inappropriate tachycardia (Figure 2.2).

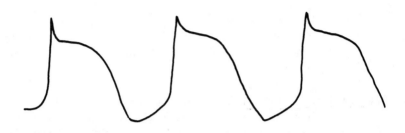

Abnormal automaticity

Figure 2.2. Abnormal automaticity causes rapid, spontaneous generation of action potentials and, thus, inappropriate tachycardia.

An antiarrhythmic drug that might be effective against automatic tachyarrhythmias is likely to reduce one or both effects. Unfortunately, no drug has been shown to reliably improve abnormal automaticity in cardiac tissue. Therefore, the mainstay of therapy is to treat the underlying illness and reverse the metabolic abnormalities causing abnormal automaticity.

Triggered Activity: Triggered arrhythmias, whether pause-dependent (i.e., caused by early afterdepolarizations [EADs]) or catechol-dependent (caused by delayed afterdepolarizations [DADs]), are related to the oscillations in the action potential. The precise mechanism of either type of afterdepolarization is only poorly understood, so no drug therapy is available that specifically eliminates the ionic fluxes responsible for EADs or DADs.

EADs are related to prolongation of the action potential in susceptible individuals. A logical treatment, therefore, is to administer a drug that reduces the duration of the action potential. Although such antiarrhythmic drugs exist (Class IB drugs), their benefit in treating triggered arrhythmias caused by EADs has been spotty at best. Instead, as mentioned in Chapter 1, the best treatments devised for EAD-mediated tachyarrhythmias have endeavored to eliminate the offending agent and to increase the heart rate to remove the pauses necessary for the development of the arrhythmias. The major significance of antiarrhythmic drugs relative to EADs is that such drugs are a common cause of EADs.

37

Similarly, the best treatment devised for DADs does not address the specific ionic causes of DADs themselves. Treating the arrhythmias most often involves discontinuing digitalis and administering beta blockers.

Reentrant Arrhythmias: In contrast to the limited usefulness of antiarrhythmic drugs in treating automatic arrhythmias and arrhythmias caused by triggered activity, antiarrhythmic drugs (in theory) directly attack the mechanism responsible for reentrant arrhythmias.

A functioning reentrant circuit requires a series of prerequisites—an anatomic or functional circuit must be present, one limb of the circuit must display slow conduction, and a second limb must display a prolonged refractory period (to produce unidirectional block). One can immediately grasp the potential benefit of a drug that, by changing the shape of the cardiac action potential, alters the conductivity and refractoriness of the tissues forming the reentrant circuit.

Figure 2.3 illustrates what might happen if a reentrant circuit were exposed to drugs. A drug that increases the duration of the cardiac action potential (thereby increasing refractory periods) further lengthens the already long refractory period of one pathway, and may thus convert unidirectional block to bidirectional block, which chemically amputates one of the pathways of the reentrant circuit. Alternatively, a drug that has the opposite effect on refractory periods—that is, it reduces the duration of the action potential and shortens refractory periods—may shorten the refrac-

Figure 2.3. Effect of antiarrhythmic drugs on a reentrant circuit. A A prototypical reentrant circuit (see Figures 1.6 and 1.7). **B** Changes that might occur with the administration of a Class III drug such as sotalol that increases the duration of the cardiac action potential and thus increases refractory periods. With such a drug, the refractory period of pathway B may be sufficiently prolonged to prevent reentry from being initiated. **C** Changes that might occur with the administration of a drug such as lidocaine that shortens the duration of the action potential and of refractory periods. The refractory period of pathway B may be shortened to the extent that the refractory periods of pathways A and B become nearly equal. A premature impulse is likely either to conduct or to block both pathways and thus prevent initiation of reentry.

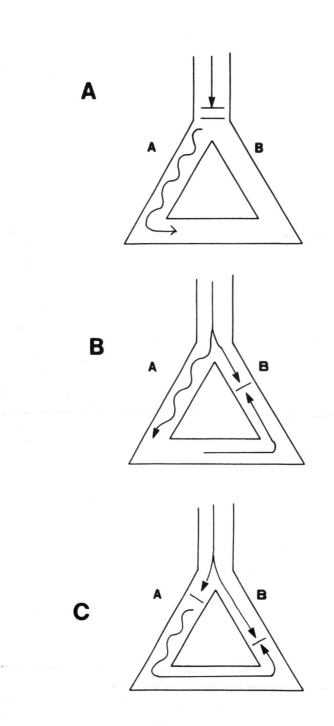

tory period of one pathway so that the refractory periods of both pathways are relatively equal. Without a difference between the refractory periods of the two limbs of the circuit, reentry cannot be initiated.

The key point in understanding how drugs affect reentrant arrhythmias is that reentry requires a critical relationship between the refractory periods and the conduction velocities of the two limbs of the reentrant circuit. Because antiarrhythmic drugs can change the refractory periods and conduction velocities, the drugs can make reentrant arrhythmias less likely to occur.

Proarrhythmia: The manner in which antiarrhythmic drugs work to benefit reentrant arrhythmias has an obvious negative implication. For example, if a patient with a previous myocardial infarction and asymptomatic nonsustained ventricular tachycardia had an occult reentrant circuit whose electrophysiologic properties were not sufficient to support a reentrant arrhythmia such as the circuit shown in Figure 2.3B, the patient might be given mexiletine to suppress the asymptomatic arrhythmia. Although it is possible that the drug will suppress the ambient ectopy, it is also possible that the mexiletine will reduce the refractory period of one pathway and give this circuit the characteristics shown in Figure 2.3A. In other words, the drug might make a reentrant arrhythmia much more likely to occur.

Anytime an antiarrhythmic drug is given to a patient with a potential reentrant circuit, the drug may make a sustained arrhythmia less likely or more likely. Both outcomes are possible; perhaps equally possible. Unfortunately, by the very same mechanism that produces an antiarrhythmic effect, antiarrhythmic drugs can also produce a proarrhythmic effect. Proarrhythmia is therefore not a bizarre, inexplicable, idiosyncratic, or rare side effect of antiarrhythmic drugs. Proarrhythmia is an entirely predictable, inherent property of antiarrhythmic drugs. Since antiarrhythmia and proarrhythmia occur by the same mechanism, one cannot have one effect without the other.

Proarrhythmia is a fairly common occurrence, but it was only poorly recognized until recently. The failure to recognize that drug therapy may worsen arrhythmias often leads to inappropriate therapy (such as increasing or adding to the offending drug) and sometimes to death. Herein lies the problem of considering antiarrhythmic drugs to be "soothing balms."

Whether an antiarrhythmic drug will make an arrhythmia better or worse is usually difficult to predict before administering the drug. Therefore, proarrhythmia is a possibility for which one must be vigilant whenever these drugs are prescribed.

CLASSIFICATION OF ANTIARRHYTHMIC DRUGS

For any set of entities, a useful classification system provides a relatively simple, logical framework that facilitates teaching and learning, aids communication, allows practical generalizations, and offers insights into the essential nature of the entities. Two general classification schemes have been set forth for antiarrhythmic drugs—the Vaughan-Williams scheme, initially proposed in 1971, and the so-called Sicilian Gambit, proposed about 20 years later. Both systems are discussed briefly below; in my opinion, the older Vaughan-Williams system more nearly fulfills the essential purpose of a classification system for the nonexpert.

Vaughan-Williams Scheme

Until the late 1960s so few antiarrhythmic drugs were available that no classification system was needed. When new drugs began to arrive with increasing frequency, however, several classification systems were proposed; the Vaughan-Williams scheme is the only one that became popular.

The Vaughan-Williams system (Table 2.1) proved useful because it groups drugs according to their major mechanism of action, that is, according to which site they bind and block on the cardiac cell membrane. Thus, Class I drugs block the sodium channel (and slow conduction velocity), Class II drugs block adrenergic receptors (and act by blunting the effect of sympathetic stimulation on cardiac electrophysiology), Class III drugs block potassium channels (and increase refractory periods), and Class IV drugs block calcium channels (and affect the areas of the heart that are depolarized primarily via calcium channels, i.e., the SA and AV nodes).

To take into account some of the obvious differences among the Class I drugs, the Vaughan-Williams system further subdivides these drugs into three subgroups: Class IA drugs—quinidine, procainamide, and disopyramide—slow conduction moderately (by slowing depolarization) and also moderately increase refractory periods (by increasing action potential duration); Class IB drugs—lidocaine, tocainide, mexiletine, phenytoin, and moricizine—do not slow conduction and actually decrease the duration of the action potential; and Class IC drugs—flecainide, encainide, and

---

Table 2.1. Vaughan-Williams Classification System of Antiarrhythmic Drugs

Class I Sodium-channel-blocking drugs
  Class IA Moderately slow conduction, moderately prolonged action potential duration
    Quinidine
    Procainamide
    Disopyramide
  Class IB Minimally slow conduction, shortened action potential duration
    Lidocaine
    Mexiletine
    Tocainide
    Phenytoin
  Class IC Markedly slow conduction, minimally prolonged action potential duration
    Flecainide
    Encainide
    Propafenone
    Moricizine
Class II Beta-blocking drugs
Class III Potassium-channel-blocking drugs
  Prolonged action potential duration
    Amiodarone
    Bretylium
    Sotalol
    Ibutilide
Class IV Calcium-channel-blocking drugs

---

propafenone—produce a pronounced slowing of conduction velocity but very little prolongation of refractory periods.

By attempting to classify drugs according to their major membrane effects, the Vaughan-Williams scheme facilitates thinking about antiarrhythmic drugs in terms of their electrophysiologic properties. The prototypical electrophysiologic effects of the various classes of drugs are depicted in Figure 2.4.

Critics of this classification system point out that antiarrhythmic drugs often cause mixed effects on the cardiac cell and that antiarrhythmic drugs in the same Vaughan-Williams group can, clinically speaking, behave quite differently from one another. The most important confounding variable relates to how antiarrhythmic drugs affect sodium and potassium channels. In fact,

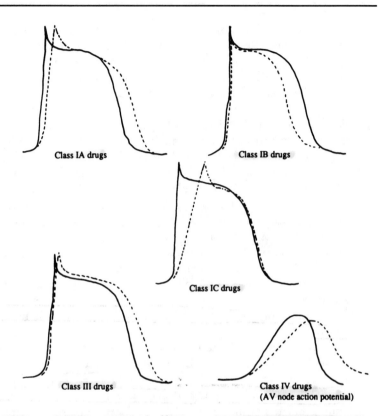

Figure 2.4. Prototypical effects on the action potential of various classes of antiarrhythmic drugs. The solid lines represent the baseline action potential; dotted lines represent the changes that result when various classes of antiarrhythmic drugs are given. The Purkinje fiber action potential is shown except in the case of Class IV drugs, for which the AV nodal action potential is depicted.

the success of the Vaughan-Williams scheme hinges, to a large extent, on its ability to characterize the variable effects of Class I and Class III drugs on the sodium and potassium channels and, thus, on conduction velocities and refractory periods.

The binding characteristics of the sodium-blocking drugs, for instance, are complex. Although all Class I drugs bind to the sodium channel, they do not bind tonically (i.e., they do not "stick" to the channel). Instead, the drugs are constantly binding and unbinding from the sodium channel. Actual blockade of the sodium channel (and thus slowing of depolarization) occurs only when a drug is bound to the sodium channel at the time the channel opens. However, many Class I drugs bind to the sodium channel only after it is already open (i.e., when it is in the "activated" state). Thus, to cause sodium channel blockade, a Class I drug first must bind to an activated sodium channel, then stay bound to that channel until the channel reopens (at which time, block finally occurs). Therefore, the effect of a Class I drug on the sodium channel depends on its binding kinetics—the rate at which that drug binds to and unbinds from the sodium channel (or alternatively, its effect depends on how "sticky" the drug is when it binds to the channel) (Figure 2.5). In the presence of "unsticky" drugs that unbind rapidly (i.e., a drug with *rapid* binding kinetics), blockade of the sodium channel may be minimal. Drugs with rapid binding kinetics therefore produce relatively little change in conduction velocity. On the other hand, "sticky" drugs that unbind slowly (i.e., drugs that have *slow* binding kinetics) produce significant blockade of the sodium channels and thus reduce conduction velocity. In general, the slower the binding kinetics of a sodium-blocking drug, the more effect the drug has on conduction velocity.

To further complicate the issue, the effect of Class I drugs on the sodium channel is partially situational. All Class I drugs, for instance, display *use dependence*: at faster heart rates, the sodium channel block increases. Use dependence is simply a result of binding kinetics, which reflects that at faster heart rates, there is time for the drug to unbind from the sodium channel before the next action potential begins; thus, at faster heart rates, the drugs have a more profound effect on conduction velocity than they have at slower heart rates. Further, ischemia, hyperkalemia, and acidosis can slow the binding kinetics of Class I drugs and thus increase the effect of the drugs on the sodium channel. For instance, lidocaine (a Class IB drug with very rapid binding kinetics and thus little effect on conduction velocity in normal tissue) can have a profound effect on ischemic tissue.

However, the Vaughan-Williams classification system does take into account the binding kinetics of the sodium-blocking drugs. Class IB drugs have very rapid sodium channel binding kinetics and, as noted, these drugs produce relatively little effect on conduction velocity. Class IC drugs have very slow binding kinetics and produce marked slowing of conduction velocity. The binding kinetics of Class IA drugs are intermediate, so these drugs have a moderate effect on conduction velocity. Thus, although no

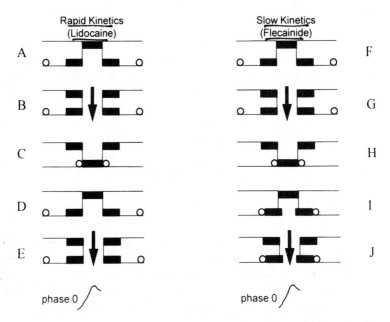

Figure 2.5. The effect of binding kinetics—the "stickiness" of a Class I drug—determines its effect on the sodium channel. As in Figure 2.1, the m and h gates are depicted; drugs are represented by open circles. Panels A through E illustrate the effect of lidocaine, a drug with rapid kinetics. A. When lidocaine is first administered, it is not yet bound to the h gate. B. The next time the cell is stimulated, the sodium channel functions normally. C. However, once the h gate becomes activated, lidocaine binds to it (many Class I drugs bind only when the binding site is in the activated state, as the h gate is in this panel). Because of the rapid unbinding of lidocaine, however, it quickly unbinds from the h gate. D. Just before the next action potential is generated, lidocaine is no longer bound. E. The next activation of the sodium channel therefore proceeds normally, and no slowing of conduction occurs. Panels F through J illustrate the effect of flecainide, a drug with slow kinetics. Panels F through H show reactions identical to those in panels A through C. G. The first activation of the sodium channel after flecainide is administered proceeds normally. H. Flecainide, like lidocaine, first binds to the h gate as soon as that gate becomes activated. Unlike lidocaine, however, flecainide displays slow unbinding kinetics. I. Just before the next action potential is generated, the drug is still attached to the h gate. J. Thus, the h gate is partially closed when the sodium channel is next engaged, which leads to slow entry of sodium into the cell, a slow upstroke in the resultant action potential, and slowing of conduction velocity. At faster heart rates, drugs such as lidocaine have less time to unbind and can behave more like flecainide.

classification system is likely to neatly characterize the nuances of sodium binding for every drug, the Vaughan-Williams system offers reasonably accurate generalizations about sodium-binding properties of antiarrhythmic drugs.

The Vaughan-Williams scheme is further challenged, however, as soon as one begins to consider the effect of antiarrhythmic drugs on the potassium channel. One of the basic premises of the Vaughan-Williams system is that Class I drugs bind the sodium channel and Class III drugs bind the potassium channel, but in fact many drugs have effects on both the sodium and potassium channels. As a result, application of the Vaughan-Williams system becomes very difficult in some cases. For instance, many experts cannot agree whether moricizine rightly belongs to Class IB or Class IC. Worse, amiodarone has properties from all four Vaughan-Williams classes. Ultimately, the classification of some drugs appears to be a matter of consensus rather than a matter of science.

Although the Vaughan-Williams scheme thus appears incapable of offering definitive classification for all possible mixtures of sodium and potassium channel blockade, it nonetheless suggests a framework for characterizing even difficult-to-classify drugs. The framework becomes apparent when one thinks of the general interplay of sodium-blocking and potassium-blocking properties as representing a continuum of possible effects instead of a categorical series of discrete effects (Figure 2.6). The advantage to thinking about drug effects along a continuum is that hard-to-classify drugs, such as moricizine and amiodarone, can be positioned at appropriate points along the continuum instead of arbitrarily being assigned to a specific class. In fact, the problem of classification is largely reduced to one of judging where on the continuum one class ends and the next begins (i.e., the problem becomes a matter of degree instead of a matter of kind). The Vaughan-Williams classification system, though admittedly imperfect, helps to locate drugs along the continuum, and therefore helps to elucidate the electrophysiologic properties even of drugs that are difficult to formally classify.

As it happens, the Vaughan-Williams scheme also allows one to make other clinically relevant generalizations about antiarrhythmic drugs. These generalizations, summarized in Table 2.2, relate to the types of arrhythmias that can be treated, the general level of efficacy and of therapy-limiting side effects, and the general risk of proarrhythmia associated with drugs within a class. (Class-

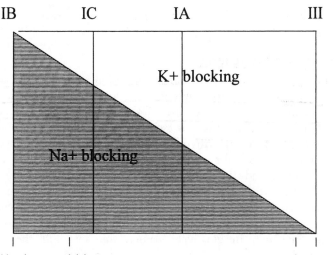

IB   IC   IA   III

K+ blocking

Na+ blocking

| | | | | |
lidocaine   moricizine   amio D-sotalol

Figure 2.6. The sodium (Na⁺)- and potassium (K⁺)-blocking properties of antiarrhythmic drugs can be displayed as a continuum of effects. Class IB drugs can be viewed as having pure sodium-blocking effects and thus hold down the left side of the grid. Class III drugs can be viewed as having pure potassium-blocking effects and thus hold down the right side of the grid. The approximate positions of the Class IC and IA drugs are illustrated. Drugs that do not quite fit the classic Vaughan-Williams classification scheme (e.g., moricizine and amiodarone) can still be positioned appropriately along the grid.

Table 2.2. Clinical Generalizations Based on Vaughan-Williams Class

Vaughan-Williams Class	Location of Activity	General Level of Efficacy	End-Organ Toxicity	Potential for Proarrhythmia
Class IA	A, V	2+	3+	2+
Class IB	V	1+	1+	1+
Class IC	A, V	3+	1+	3+
Class II	AVN, V	1+	1+	0
Class III	A, V	2+ (amio 4+)	1+ (amio 4+)	2+ (amio 1+)
Class IV	AVN	1+	1+	0

A = atrium; amio = amiodarone; AVN = atrioventricular node; V = ventricle.

specific features of antiarrhythmic drugs are discussed in Part 2 of the book.)

Sicilian Gambit Scheme

In 1990, a group of eminent electrophysiologists retreated to Taormina, Sicily, to consider the issue of the classification of antiarrhythmic drugs because of the well-recognized limitations of the Vaughan-Williams scheme: the oversimplification of concepts about antiarrhythmic drugs, the common grouping of drugs with dissimilar actions, the inability to group certain drugs accurately, and the failure to take into account many actions of antiarrhythmic drugs that became recognized long after the Vaughan-Williams system had been proposed. What emerged was a new approach to the classification of antiarrhythmic drugs; the inventors imaginatively named the approach the Sicilian Gambit.

The Vaughan-Williams scheme is based on whether drugs produce block in one or more of a few sites on the cell membrane, but the Sicilian Gambit takes into account a host of additional actions of antiarrhythmic drugs—the type and degree of blockade of channels, antagonistic and agonistic effects on receptors, effects on the sodium–potassium pump, the time constants of binding to cellular sites, effects on second messengers, and the affinity for binding on the basis of whether the cell is in an active or inactive state. The resultant schema is shown in Figure 2.7.

Two major differences exist between the Vaughan-Williams scheme and the Sicilian Gambit approach. First, the Sicilian Gambit is far more thorough than the Vaughan-Williams system in describing the precise actions of antiarrhythmic drugs. Second, inasmuch as each drug is essentially in its own class (since no two drugs are exactly alike in all the ways listed), the Sicilian Gambit is not a true classification system. Instead, it is a tabular list of virtually everything known about each drug.

This is not to say that the Sicilian Gambit is not useful. It is, in fact, useful to have a complete tabulation of drug effects. Such a table allows one to easily compare the recognized similarities and differences between drugs. Further, when the mechanisms of arrhythmias have become more precisely delineated, a precise knowledge of individual drugs may help in formulating more accurate guesses as to effective pharmacologic therapy (which was a specific goal in devising the Sicilian Gambit) although it is likely to be always true that nearly identical patients with nearly identical

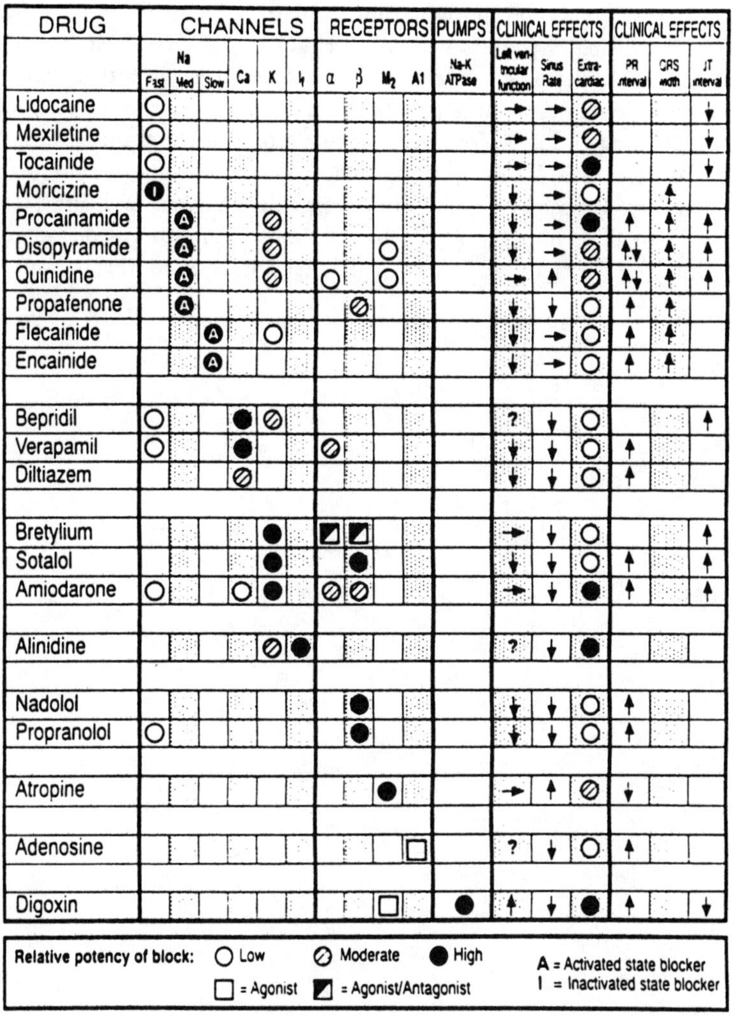

DRUG	CHANNELS Na Fast	Na Med	Na Slow	Ca	K	If	RECEPTORS α	β	M₂	A1	PUMPS Na-K ATPase	CLINICAL EFFECTS Left ventricular function	Sinus Rate	Extra-cardiac	CLINICAL EFFECTS PR interval	QRS width	JT interval
Lidocaine	○											→	→	⊘			↓
Mexiletine	○											→	→	⊘			↓
Tocainide	○											→	→	●			↓
Moricizine	● I											↓	→	○		↑	
Procainamide		Ⓐ			⊘							↓	→	●	↑	↑	↑
Disopyramide		Ⓐ			⊘				○			↓	→	⊘	↑↓	↑	↑
Quinidine		Ⓐ			⊘		○		○			→	↑	⊘	↑↓	↑	↑
Propafenone		Ⓐ						⊘				↓	↓	○	↑	↑	
Flecainide			Ⓐ		○							↓	→	○	↑	↑	
Encainide			Ⓐ									↓	→	○	↑	↑	
Bepridil	○			●	⊘							?	↓	○			↑
Verapamil	○			●			⊘					↓	↓	○	↑		
Diltiazem				⊘								↓	↓	○	↑		
Bretylium					●		▨	▨				→	↓	○			↑
Sotalol					●			●				↓	↓	○	↑		↑
Amiodarone	○			○	●		⊘	⊘				→	↓	●	↑	↑	↑
Alinidine					⊘	●						?	↓	●			
Nadolol								●				↓	↓	○	↑		
Propranolol	○							●				↓	↓	○	↑		
Atropine									●			→	↑	⊘	↓		
Adenosine										□		?	↓	○	↑		
Digoxin										□	●	↑	↓	●	↑		↓

Relative potency of block: ○ Low ⊘ Moderate ● High □ = Agonist ▨ = Agonist/Antagonist

A = Activated state blocker
I = Inactivated state blocker

Figure 2.7. The Sicilian Gambit, a schema listing all major known properties of antiarrhythmic drugs. Effects of each drug on channels, receptors, and pumps are shown, as are some of the clinical effects. (Reproduced with permission from Members of the Sicilian Gambit. *Antiarrhythmic Therapy: A Pathophysiologic Approach.* Armonk, NY: Futura, 1994:94.)

arrhythmias often respond differently to the same drug. In addition, a tabulated system is certainly helpful to basic researchers.

However, because the Sicilian Gambit is not a true classification system, it does not offer much help to the nonexpert in learning about or communicating about antiarrhythmic drugs. Nor does it aid in formulating practical generalizations about these drugs. Especially for the nonexpert, the Vaughan-Williams system, with all its limitations, remains the most useful means of categorizing antiarrhythmic drugs; it is the system used throughout this book.

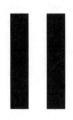

Clinical Features of Antiarrhythmic Drugs

Class I Antiarrhythmic Drugs

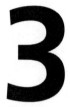

The feature that gains an antiarrhythmic drug admission into Class I is blockade of the rapid sodium channel. Yet, because of the varied effects on the sodium channel and the potassium channel, drugs assigned to Class I can behave very differently from one another. On the basis of their sodium and potassium effects, Class I drugs have been subclassified into groups IA, IB, and IC. The major clinical features, electrophysiologic properties, and adverse effects of Class I antiarrhythmic drugs are summarized in the accompanying tables.

CLASS IA

Class IA drugs can be thought of as all-purpose antiarrhythmic agents because they are moderately effective in treating most types of tachyarrhythmias. Unfortunately, they are also moderately effective in causing both major varieties of side effects—end-organ effects and proarrhythmic effects.

As shown in Figure 3.1, Class IA drugs block the rapid sodium channel (slowing the upstroke of the cardiac action potential and slowing conduction velocity) and the potassium channel (prolonging the duration of the action potential and prolonging refractoriness). These electrophysiologic effects are manifested in both atrial and ventricular tissue, and therefore Class IA drugs have the potential of benefiting both atrial and ventricular tachyarrhythmias. The major clinical features of Class IA antiarrhythmic drugs are summarized in Table 3.1, and the major electrophysiologic features are summarized in Table 3.2.

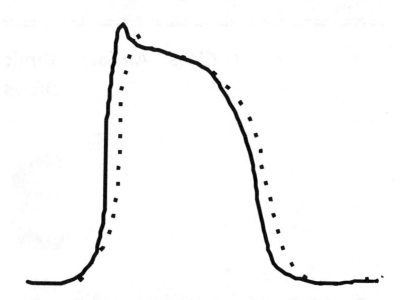

Figure 3.1. **Effect of Class IA drugs on the cardiac action potential. Baseline action potential is displayed as a solid line; the dashed line indicates the effect of Class IA drugs.**

Table 3.1. Clinical Pharmacology of Class IA Drugs

	Quinidine	Procainamide	Disopyramide
GI absorption	80–90%	70–90%	80–90%
Protein binding	80–90%	Weak	Variable (less binding at higher drug levels)
Elimination	Liver	Metabolized in liver to NAPA; PA and NAPA excreted by kidneys	60% kidneys 40% liver
Half-life	5–8 hr	3–5 hr	8–9 hr
Therapeutic level	2–5 μg/mL	4–12 μg/mL (PA) 9–20 μg/mL (NAPA)	2–5 μg/mL
Dosage range	300–600 mg q6hr (sulfate) 324–972 mg q6–8hr (gluconate)	15 mg/kg IV, then 1–6 mg/min IV; or 500–1250 mg PO q6hr	100–200 mg q6hr

NAPA = *N*-acetylprocainamide; PA = procainamide.

Table 3.2. Electrophysiologic Effects of Class IA Drugs

	Quinidine	Procainamide	Disopyramide
Conduction velocity	Decrease ++	Decrease ++	Decrease ++
Refractory periods	Increase ++	Increase ++	Increase ++
Automaticity	Suppress +	Suppress +	Suppress +
Afterdepolarizations	May cause EADs	May cause EADs	May cause EADs
Efficacy			
Atrial fib/flutter	++	++	++
AVN reentry	+	+	+
Macroreentry	+	+	+
PVCs	++	++	++
VT/VF	++	++	++

AVN = AV node; EADs = early afterdepolarizations; PVCs = premature ventricular complexes; VT/VF = ventricular tachycardia and ventricular fibrillation.

Quinidine

Quinidine is the D-isomer of the antimalarial quinine, a drug that was noted to be effective in the treatment of palpitations as long ago as the eighteenth century. Quinidine itself was recognized as an effective antiarrhythmic agent in the early twentieth century, and remains a frequently used agent.

Clinical Pharmacology: Quinidine is administered orally as one of three salts (quinidine sulfate, quinidine gluconate, or quinidine polygalacturonate). Three formulations have been marketed because some patients tolerate one salt better than another. Approximately 80% to 90% of the sulfate preparation is absorbed, and peak plasma concentrations are reached within 2 hours. The gluconate and polygalacturonate preparations are absorbed more slowly and less completely than the sulfate formulation. Quinidine is 80% to 90% protein bound in the circulation, and has a large volume of distribution. The concentration of the drug is 4 to 10 times higher in the heart, liver, and kidneys than it is in the circulation. The drug is eliminated mainly through hepatic metabolism. Its elimination half-life is 5 to 8 hours but may be prolonged in patients with congestive heart failure or in the elderly.

Electrophysiologic Effects: Quinidine blocks the sodium channel and slows the rate of depolarization of the action potential. Like all Class IA drugs, quinidine binds and unbinds from the sodium channel more slowly than does lidocaine, but more rapidly than do Class IC agents. Thus, its effect on conduction velocity is midway between drugs in Class IB and IC. Its effects on the potassium channels result in prolongation of the action potential and, therefore, of the refractory period. The electrophysiologic effects are seen in both atrial and ventricular tissues. Quinidine can suppress automaticity in Purkinje fibers. Like all drugs that prolong refractoriness, quinidine can cause early afterdepolarizations (and thus torsades de pointes) in susceptible individuals.

Hemodynamic Effects: Quinidine blocks the α-adrenergic receptors, which can lead to peripheral vasodilation and reflex sinus tachycardia. The effects tend to be minimal when the drug is given orally but can be profound with intravenous administration. (Thus, the intravenous form of quinidine is used only rarely.) Quinidine also has a vagolytic effect, which can manifest by improving conduction through the AV node. The vagolytic effect is important clinically when one is treating atrial fibrillation or flutter—enhanced AV nodal conduction can lead to increases in ventricular response when quinidine is administered without also administering AV nodal-blocking agents. No significant myocardial depression occurs with quinidine.

Therapeutic Uses: Quinidine is moderately effective in treating both atrial and ventricular tachyarrhythmias. Approximately 50% of patients treated with quinidine for atrial fibrillation remain in sinus rhythm after 1 year. Quinidine acts on the accessory pathway in patients with bypass-tract-mediated tachycardias and on the fast pathway in patients with AV nodal reentrant tachycardia. Thus, quinidine has been used to treat all types of reentrant supraventricular tachyarrhythmias.

Quinidine is effective in suppressing premature ventricular complexes and nonsustained ventricular tachycardias, but because of the proarrhythmic potential of quinidine (and most other antiarrhythmic agents), these arrhythmias should not be treated except to suppress significant symptoms. When guided by serial drug testing in the electrophysiology laboratory, quinidine is effective 15% to 25% of the time in suppressing inducible sustained ventricular tachycardia. Again, because of the drug's proarrhythmic potential, quinidine should not be used to treat sustained ventricular tachycardia without the guidance of electrophysiologic testing (or without the protection of an implantable defibrillator).

Adverse Effects and Interactions: Symptomatic side effects occur in 30% to 50% of patients taking quinidine, and the drug must be discontinued in 20% to 30% of patients because of toxicity. The most common side effects are gastrointestinal, mainly diarrhea. In general, if diarrhea occurs, the drug should be discontinued— because the diarrhea is usually not adequately controlled with medication, the resultant electrolyte imbalances may exacerbate the arrhythmias that one is attempting to suppress. Quinidine can also cause dizziness, headache, or cinchonism (tinnitus, visual blurring, hearing disturbances). Rashes are fairly common, and significant hypersensitivity reactions such as hemolytic anemia and thrombocytopenia can also occur. Lupus and hepatitis have been reported.

As is the case with all Class IA drugs, proarrhythmia is a major consideration when one elects to use quinidine. Any drug that prolongs the duration of the action potential can produce torsades de pointes in susceptible individuals, and any drug that alters conduction velocity or refractoriness can exacerbate reentrant arrhythmias. Quinidine thus can (and does) cause ventricular arrhythmias by either mechanism. Quinidine syncope was recognized decades ago, but it was only relatively recently that this clinical syndrome was shown to be caused by ventricular tachyarrhythmias. Quinidine-induced ventricular arrhythmias tend to occur early, most often within 3 to 5 days of the beginning of therapy, but can occur at any time. Although the magnitude of quinidine-induced proarrhythmia is difficult to quantify, a meta-analysis of randomized trials using quinidine to treat atrial fibrillation indicated a total mortality of 2.9% in patients receiving quinidine, compared with a mortality of 0.8% in patients receiving placebo. The excess mortality may be mainly a result of proarrhythmia. This sort of evidence strongly suggests that patients should be placed on a cardiac monitor for several days when treatment with quinidine is elected.

Several relevant drug interactions have been reported with quinidine. Quinidine potentiates the effect of anticholinergics, warfarin, and phenothiazines. Increased digoxin levels routinely occur when quinidine is given to patients taking digoxin. Quinidine levels are decreased by phenobarbital, rifampin, and phenytoin; they are increased by amiodarone.

Procainamide

Procainamide came into clinical use in 1951. Its availability in both oral and intravenous forms has made it an attractive drug for treating both acute and chronic tachyarrhythmias.

Clinical Pharmacology: When given intravenously, procainamide's onset of action is almost immediate; after oral intake, the onset of action is approximately 1 hour. Absorption after oral intake is 70% to 90%, and the drug is only weakly protein bound. Fifty percent of the drug is excreted in the urine, and variable amounts of procainamide are metabolized by the liver to N-acetylprocainamide (NAPA), an active metabolite with Class III properties. The amount of NAPA in the plasma depends on hepatic function and the acetylator phenotype (approximately 50% of the population are "slow acetylators," and these individuals may be more susceptible to procainamide-induced lupus). Both the parent compound and NAPA are excreted by the kidneys. The elimination half-life is 3 to 5 hours in normal individuals. Assays for measuring plasma levels of both procainamide and NAPA are readily available.

Dosage: Intravenous loading of procainamide should be given no more rapidly than 50 mg/min to minimize hemodynamic side effects to a total dose of 15 mg/kg. Administration should be slowed if hypotension occurs, and should be stopped if the QRS interval increases by more than 50% or if heart block occurs. A maintenance infusion of 1–6 mg/min can be used to maintain therapeutic levels. By oral administration, 3–6 g/day are usually given. With currently available long-acting preparations, procainamide can be given every 6 to 12 hours. Because of its short half-life, administration every 3 to 4 hours is required with standard preparations.

Electrophysiologic Effects: The electrophysiologic effects of procainamide are similar to those of quinidine.

Hemodynamic Effects: Similar to quinidine, procainamide causes arteriolar vasodilation, an effect that is seen almost exclusively when the drug is given intravenously. The effect is easier to control with procainamide than with quinidine by infusing the drug slowly, which explains why clinicians are less reluctant to administer intravenous procainamide than quinidine. Procainamide has some anticholinergic effect, but less than that of quinidine. Negative inotropic effects are negligible, except when toxic levels of the drug are reached, especially when NAPA levels exceed 30 µg/mL.

Therapeutic Uses: The therapeutic uses of procainamide are similar to those of quinidine. The drug can be used for all varieties of reentrant atrial and ventricular arrhythmias, and its overall efficacy for both atrial and ventricular tachyarrhythmias is similar to that of quinidine. Because procainamide is available for relatively rapid intravenous loading, it is the drug of choice for treating atrial fibrillation with rapid conduction down a bypass tract, although nondrug therapy—direct current (DC) cardioversion—works instantaneously in this condition. Procainamide is also used commonly for the acute conversion of atrial fibrillation and atrial flutter and to terminate or slow incessant ventricular tachycardias.

Adverse Effects and Interactions: Early side effects with procainamide include hypotension when the drug is administered intravenously and gastrointestinal problems (especially nausea, vomiting, and diarrhea) in as much as 25% of patients treated. With chronic administration of procainamide, agranulocytosis is the most serious problem. The problem is rare, but carries a mortality as high as 25%. Agranulocytosis is usually seen within the first 3 months of therapy. Drug-induced lupus occurs in 20% of patients who take the drug chronically and may be manifested by fever, rash, arthritis, pleuritis, or pericarditis. Symptoms usually resolve within a few weeks of discontinuing the drug.

Procainamide levels may be increased when the drug is given with amiodarone, trimethoprim, and especially cimetidine (but not ranitidine). Alcohol can decrease procainamide levels by increasing hepatic metabolism.

The cautions relative to proarrhythmia are the same for procainamide as those for quinidine.

Disopyramide

Disopyramide is chemically dissimilar to quinidine and procainamide but has virtually the same electrophysiologic effects. Disopyramide was approved by the United States Food and Drug Administration (FDA) in 1977.

Clinical Pharmacology: Disopyramide is an oral agent. Absorption is high (80% to 90%), and peak blood levels occur 2 to 3 hours after administration. Protein binding of the drug depends on plasma concentration—at higher levels, less of the drug is bound; thus, toxicity is especially significant at higher drug levels. Approximately 60% of the drug is excreted by the kidneys, and 40% is metabolized in the liver. Its major metabolite (an alkylated compound) has significant anticholinergic properties. The elimination half-life is 8 to 9 hours in normal individuals.

Dosage: The usual dosage of disopyramide is 100–200 mg every 6 hours. A longer-acting form given 200–300 mg every 12 hours is now available. The dosage should be adjusted downward in the presence of either hepatic or renal insufficiency.

Electrophysiologic Effects: The electrophysiologic effects of disopyramide are similar to those of quinidine. In addition, disopyramide has significant anticholinergic effects, which can increase the sinus rate and enhance AV nodal conduction.

Hemodynamic Effects: Disopyramide has a strong negative inotropic effect and should not be used in patients with depressed myocardial function, especially in patients with a history of congestive heart failure (more than 50% of whom have acute hemodynamic decompensation after administration of disopyramide).

Therapeutic Uses: The therapeutic profile of disopyramide is very similar to that of quinidine. Its clinical usefulness, however, has been limited by its negative inotropic potential and its relatively strong anticholinergic properties. Aside from treating arrhythmias, disopyramide also has been reported to be effective in some patients with cardioneurogenic (vasovagal) syncope, presumably because its negative inotropic effects can delay the recruitment of cardiac C fibers (one of the afferent pathways that can stimulate the vasodepressor region of the medulla).

Adverse Effects and Interactions: The major adverse effects of disopyramide are related to myocardial depression and anticholinergic side effects. Disopyramide should not be used in patients with significant ventricular dysfunction, especially if they have a history of congestive heart failure. Symptoms of dry mouth, eyes, nose, and throat occur in as much as 40% of patients taking disopyramide. Urinary difficulty or urinary retention are significant problems with disopyramide in men older than 50 years but can also be seen in women. The drug can precipitate closed-angle glaucoma and should not be used in patients with a family history of glaucoma.

Proarrhythmic effects of disopyramide are similar to those of quinidine.

Drug interactions include the decreasing of plasma disopyramide levels by phenobarbital, phenytoin, and rifampin. Other drugs with negative inotropic effects can exacerbate the myocardial depression seen with disopyramide.

CLASS IB

Class IB drugs are moderately useful in treating ventricular arrhythmias. Their major advantage is that, in marked contrast to the other Class I drugs, they have a low potential for causing proarrhythmia.

As shown in Figure 3.2, Class IB drugs have relatively little effect on the rapid sodium channel at normal heart rates and at

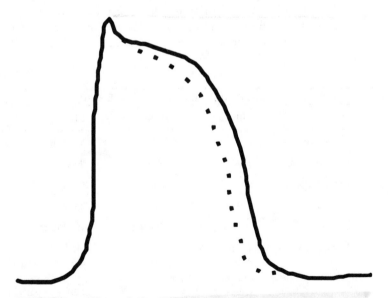

Figure 3.2. Effect of Class IB drugs on the cardiac action potential. Baseline action potential is displayed as a solid line; the dashed line indicates the effect of Class IB drugs.

therapeutic serum concentrations, so they have little effect on conduction velocity. Their effect is to decrease the duration of the action potential, and therefore these drugs tend to decrease refractory periods. Probably because the duration of the action potential in atrial tissue is already shorter than that of ventricular tissue, Class IB drugs have little effect on atrial tissue and thus are useful only in the treatment of ventricular arrhythmias. Tables 3.3 and 3.4 summarize the major clinical features and electrophysiologic properties of Class IB antiarrhythmic drugs.

Lidocaine

Lidocaine has been used clinically since 1943 when it was introduced as a local anesthetic agent. In the 1950s, it gradually came into use for the acute treatment of ventricular arrhythmias, and it remains the drug of first choice for ventricular arrhythmias in many acute situations.

Clinical Pharmacology: Although lidocaine is well absorbed in the gut, it is subject to extensive first-pass metabolism in the liver, so it is normally administered intravenously. Very little of the drug is excreted by the kidneys even after intravenous administration. Lidocaine is 70% bound to protein in plasma. Further, the proteins that bind lidocaine are acute-phase reactants; that is, during periods of stress, such as acute myocardial infarction, the proteins that bind

Table 3.3. Clinical Pharmacology of Class IB Drugs

	Lidocaine	Mexiletine	Phenytoin
GI absorption	—	>90%	Variable
Protein binding	70%	70%	90%
Elimination	Liver	Liver	Liver
Half-life	1–4 hr	8–16 hr	24 hr
Therapeutic level	1.5–5 µg/mL	0.75–2 µg/mL	10–20 µg/mL
Dosage range	1.5 mg/kg IV, then 1–4 mg/min; repeat $^1/_2$ initial dose after 10 min	150–200 mg q8hr	Oral: 300–500 mg/day in divided doses; IV loading: 7.5–10 mg at rate of 50 mg every 2 min

Table 3.4. Electrophysiologic Effects of Class IB Drugs

	Lidocaine	Mexiletine	Phenytoin
Conduction velocity	−	−	−
Refractory periods	Decrease	Decrease	Decrease
	+	+	+
Automaticity	Suppress	Suppress	Suppress
	+ +	+ ,	+
Afterdepolarizations	Suppresses EADs and DADs	Suppresses DADs	Suppresses DADs
	+	+	+ +
Efficacy			
Atrial fib/flutter	−	−	−
AVN reentry	−	−	−
Macroreentry	+/−	−	−
PVCs	+ +	+ +	+
VT/VF	+	+	+

AVN = AV node; EADs = early afterdepolarizations; DADs = delayed afterdepolarizations; PVCs = premature ventricular complexes; VT/VF = ventricular tachycardia and ventricular fibrillation.

lidocaine increase in plasma. Increased plasma binding during stress can cause lidocaine levels to increase during a constant infusion and prolong the elimination half-life from 1 or 2 hours to as long as 4 hours.

Dosage: Lidocaine is generally loaded acutely by giving 1.5 mg/kg intravenously and initiating a constant infusion of 1–4 mg/min. When lidocaine is given acutely, it is rapidly distributed to the target organs (phase I distribution), but within 20 minutes is distributed throughout the rest of the body (phase II distribution); the initial immediate efficacy of the drug falls off during phase II. Thus, two or three additional boluses are usually given at 10-minute intervals after the original bolus—the dosage of the additional boluses is usually half that of the initial bolus.

Electrophysiologic Effects: Typical of Class IB drugs, lidocaine (mainly because of its rapid-binding kinetics) causes no slowing of the depolarization phase of the action potential and no slowing in conduction velocity in normal tissue. However, at fast heart rates or during ischemia, hypokalemia, or acidosis, lidocaine can substantially slow depolarization and conduction velocity. The duration of the action potential and the duration of refractoriness is shortened by lidocaine in ventricular tissue but not in atrial tissue. Lidocaine can suppress both normal and abnormal automaticity, which can lead to asystole when lidocaine is given in the setting of a ventricular escape rhythm. Lidocaine can also suppress early and late afterdepolarizations.

Hemodynamic Effects: Lidocaine has little or no hemodynamic effect.

Therapeutic Uses: Lidocaine is effective for ventricular tachyarrhythmias and is usually the drug of choice for the emergent therapy of such arrhythmias because therapeutic plasma levels can be obtained rapidly. The drug has been shown to decrease the incidence of ventricular fibrillation in the setting of acute myocardial infarction but does not improve mortality. In fact, recent data suggest that the routine prophylactic use of lidocaine in acute infarction when the patient has arrived in the hospital may actually increase mortality.

Adverse Effects and Interactions: The predominant side effects relate to the central nervous system. Slurred speech, dizziness, perioral numbness and paresthesias, seizures, and respiratory arrest can all occur and are generally associated with toxic plasma levels.

Other drugs may affect plasma levels of lidocaine. Propranolol, metoprolol, and cimetidine (but not ranitidine) decrease hepatic blood flow and result in increased levels of lidocaine. Phenobarbital decreases plasma concentrations of lidocaine.

Lidocaine causes proarrhythmia only rarely.

Mexiletine

Mexiletine is an orally administered congener of lidocaine and was approved by the FDA in 1986.

Clinical Pharmacology: Mexiletine is nearly completely absorbed from the gut and displays minimal first-pass hepatic clearance. Peak plasma levels occur in 4 to 6 hours, and the drug is approximately 70% protein bound. The drug is mainly metabolized by the liver, and the elimination half-life has been reported to be from 8 to 16 hours.

Dosage: Because of the variable metabolism and because therapeutic and toxic doses of mexiletine tend to overlap, dosage must be individualized. Generally, unless hepatic disease is present, 150 mg is given every 8 hours. If there is no response after several days (at least 3 days) and if toxicity is not present, dosage can be increased to 200 mg every 8 hours. Dosage can be further increased after several more days unless toxicity is present, but rarely can more than 750 mg/day be administered without significant side effects.

Electrophysiologic Effects: The electrophysiologic effects of mexiletine are virtually identical to those of lidocaine.

Hemodynamic Effects: Mexiletine has little or no effect on blood pressure or cardiac function.

Therapeutic Uses: The therapeutic profile of mexiletine is similar to that of lidocaine; that is, it effectively suppresses ventricular arrhythmias. Unlike lidocaine, however, mexiletine is not particularly suitable for the treatment of emergent or acute arrhythmias because titrating the drug to an effective dose may take many days. Its use has thus been limited to treating chronic ventricular arrhythmias. Although mexiletine is effective in suppressing premature ventricular complexes and nonsustained ventricular tachycardia, these arrhythmias should generally not be treated unless they are producing significant symptoms. On the basis of serial drug testing in the electrophysiology laboratory, mexiletine rarely suppresses inducible sustained ventricular tachycardia; the drug is estimated to be effective for such suppression in only 5% to 10% of patients tested.

Adverse Effects and Interactions: As with lidocaine, central nervous system side effects predominate—tremor, blurred vision, and ataxia are the most common effects. Gastrointestinal symptoms are also common.

Mexiletine levels can be lowered by phenytoin, phenobarbitol, and rifampin. Mexiletine levels can be increased by cimetidine, chloramphenicol, and isoniazid. Theophylline levels can be increased substantially when the drug is given with mexiletine. The side effects of mexiletine and lidocaine can be additive.

Typical of Class IB antiarrhythmic drugs, mexiletine displays only rare proarrhythmic effects.

Tocainide

Tocainide is another oral analogue of lidocaine. Its properties are very similar to mexiletine, except that it is eliminated from the system by both the liver and the kidneys. Because tocainide was found to cause agranulocytosis in a small but substantial subset of patients exposed to the drug, it is essentially no longer used clinically except for the very rare patient who needs a Class IB drug chronically but who cannot tolerate other drugs in this class.

Phenytoin

Phenytoin came into clinical use as an anticonvulsant in 1938. By the early 1950s, the drug was recognized to have antiarrhythmic properties. The drug enjoyed brief popularity as an antiarrhythmic agent in the early 1960s, but was almost entirely supplanted when lidocaine and procainamide came into widespread use. Phenytoin has never been approved by the FDA for treating cardiac arrhythmias. In general, phenytoin is not widely thought of as an antiarrhythmic agent, but it can occasionally be quite useful for this purpose.

Clinical Pharmacology: Phenytoin's oral absorption is relatively slow and highly variable. Peak serum levels can occur from 3 to 12 hours after an oral dose. The drug is 90% protein bound, and is metabolized by the liver to inactive compounds. At lower plasma levels ($<10\,\mu g/mL$), elimination is exponential. At higher plasma levels, elimination is dose dependent, and plasma levels increase disproportionately as dosage is increased. The average elimination half-life is 24 hours, but this value is highly variable.

Dosage: A drug-loading regimen is usually recommended with oral administration of phenytoin, especially if therapeutic levels are desired within 24 hours. Generally, 15 mg/kg is given orally in divided doses on day 1, followed by 7.5 mg/kg on day 2, followed by a maintenance dosage of 5 mg/kg on subsequent days (usually 300–500 mg/day in two or three divided doses). Chronic dosage should not be changed more often than at 10- to 14-day intervals because of the dose-dependent elimination of the drug.

Phenytoin can also be administered intravenously, preferably through a central intravenous line because of the tendency to produce phlebitis. As much as 50 mg/min can be given intravenously to a total dose of 7.5–10 mg/kg. Monitoring for the appearance of lateral gaze nystagmus during administration of the drug can be a useful indicator of therapeutic serum levels (10–20 µg/mL).

Electrophysiologic Effects: The electrophysiologic profile of phenytoin is similar to that of lidocaine—it displays a rate-dependent effect on the sodium channel with rapid binding-unbinding characteristics. Thus, conduction velocity is minimally affected in normal tissue and at normal heart rates. Unlike other Class IB drugs, phenytoin also displays a centrally mediated antiadrenergic effect. Delayed afterdepolarizations of the type seen with digitalis toxicity are suppressed by phenytoin.

Hemodynamic Effects: With rapid intravenous loading, hypotension can occur but can be controlled by titrating the rate of drug administration. Hypotension does not occur with oral administration. Phenytoin has no negative inotropic effects.

Therapeutic Uses: Phenytoin is effective for ventricular tachyarrhythmias that occur with digitalis toxicity, most likely because it suppresses delayed afterdepolarizations. In addition, because of its Class IB effects, phenytoin is occasionally effective in suppressing inducible sustained ventricular tachycardias in the electrophysiology laboratory (10% to 12% of the time). Phenytoin has also been moderately effective in suppressing ventricular arrhythmias in intensive care unit (ICU) settings in which enhanced automaticity is often invoked as an arrhythmic mechanism (ICU arrhythmias).

Adverse Effects and Interactions: The most common side effects involve the gastrointestinal and central nervous systems. Central nervous system symptoms (mainly ataxia and nystagmus) are related to plasma levels. Other less common side effects include osteomalacia (from interference with vitamin D metabolism), megaloblastic anemia (from interference with folate metabolism), and hypersensitivity reactions such as lupus, hepatic necrosis, hematologic disorders, and pseudolymphoma. Gingival hyperplasia, said to occur in as much as 20% of children taking phenytoin, appears to be relatively rare in adults.

Several drug interactions have been seen with phenytoin. Phenytoin increases plasma levels of theophylline, quinidine, disopyramide, lidocaine, and mexiletine. Phenytoin levels are increased by cimetidine, isoniazid, sulfonamides, and amiodarone. Plasma levels of phenytoin can be reduced by theophylline.

Like other Class IB drugs, phenytoin rarely causes proarrhythmia.

CLASS IC

Class IC drugs generated much excitement in the early to late 1980s because they are very effective in treating both atrial and ventricular tachyarrhythmias and generally cause only mild end-organ toxicity. When the proarrhythmic potential of Class IC drugs was more fully appreciated, however, the drugs quickly fell out of favor, and one (encainide) was taken off the market.

As shown in Figure 3.3, Class IC drugs have a relatively pronounced effect on the rapid sodium channel because of their slow sodium-channel-binding kinetics. Thus, they significantly slow conduction velocity even at normal heart rates. They have only a modest effect on repolarization. Class IC drugs have similar effects on both atrial and ventricular tissue and are useful for both atrial and ventricular tachyarrhythmias. The major clinical features of Class IC antiarrhythmic drugs are summarized in Table 3.5, and the major electrophysiologic properties are shown in Table 3.6.

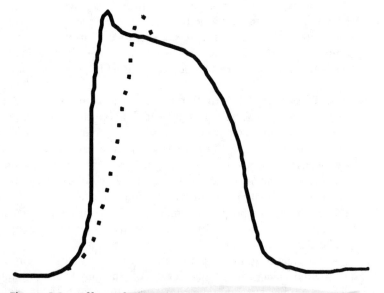

Figure 3.3. Effect of Class IC drugs on the cardiac action potential. Baseline action potential is displayed as a solid line; the dashed line indicates the effect of Class IC drugs.

Table 3.5. Clinical Pharmacology of Class IC Drugs

	Flecainide	Propafenone	Moricizine
GI absorption	>90%	>90%	>90%
Protein binding	40%	90%	>90%
Elimination	70% liver 30% kidneys	Liver	Liver (metabolized to >2 doz compounds)
Half-life	12–24 hr	6–7 hr	Variable; usually 3–12 hr
Therapeutic level	0.2–1 µg/mL	0.2–1 µg/mL	—
Dosage range	100–200 mg q12hr	150–300 mg q8hr	200–300 mg q8hr

Table 3.6. Electrophysiologic Effects of Class IC Drugs

	Flecainide	Propafenone	Moricizine
Conduction velocity	Decrease +++	Decrease +++	Decrease ++
Refractory periods	No change (may lengthen RP in atrium)	No change	Decrease +
Automaticity	−	Suppresses +	Suppresses +
Afterdepolarizations	−	−	Suppresses EADs and DADs +
Efficacy			
Atrial fib/flutter	++	++	+
AVN reentry	++	++	+
Macroreentry	++	++	+
PVCs	+++	+++	++
VT/VF	++	++	++

AVN = AV node; EADs = early afterdepolarizations; DADs = delayed after-depolarizations; RP = refractory periods; PVCs = premature ventricular complexes; VT/VF = ventricular tachycardia and ventricular fibrillation.

Flecainide

Flecainide was synthesized in 1972 and approved by the FDA in 1984.

Clinical Pharmacology: Flecainide is well absorbed from the gastrointestinal tract, and peak plasma levels are reached 2 to 4 hours after an oral dose. Forty percent of the drug is protein bound. The drug is mainly metabolized by the liver (70%), but 30% is excreted unchanged by the kidneys. Flecainide has a long elimination half-life (12 to 24 hr), so a steady state is not reached for 3 to 5 days after a change in oral dosage.

Dosage: The usual dosage is 100–400 mg/day orally, in divided doses. Generally, the beginning dosage is 100 mg every 12 hours. Dosage can be increased by 50 mg/dose (at 3- to 5-day intervals) to a maximal dosage of 200 mg every 12 hours.

Electrophysiologic Effects: The major electrophysiologic feature of flecainide is a substantial slowing in conduction velocity. The prolonged slowing is directly related to the prolonged binding-unbinding time (i.e., the slow-binding kinetics) of the drug. Although most Class IA agents have binding times in the range of 5 seconds, and Class IB drugs have binding times of approximately 0.3 seconds, flecainide has a binding time of 30 seconds. Thus, flecainide is virtually continuously bound to the sodium channel, and therefore produces slow conduction even at low heart rates (i.e., at rest). Flecainide subsequently has a dose-dependent effect on the electrocardiogram, manifested by a progressive prolongation of the PR and QRS intervals, with only a minor effect on the QT interval. The drug depresses conduction in all areas of the heart.

Hemodynamic Effects: Flecainide has a pronounced negative inotropic effect similar to that of disopyramide. The drug should probably not be given to patients with a history of congestive heart failure or with significantly depressed left ventricular ejection fraction.

Therapeutic Uses: As one might predict from the universal nature of the drug's electrophysiologic properties, flecainide has an effect on both atrial and ventricular tachyarrhythmias. It has been shown to be effective for terminating and preventing atrial fibrillation and atrial flutter; if the arrhythmias recur, flecainide can slow the ventricular response. Because it affects accessory pathway function, flecainide is useful in the treatment of bypass-tract-mediated tachyarrhythmias. The drug has a profound suppressive effect on premature ventricular complexes and nonsustained ventricular tachycardia. It has been reported to suppress approximately 20% to 25% of inducible sustained ventricular tachycardias in the electrophysiology laboratory.

Flecainide is unsurpassed in suppressing premature ventricular complexes and nonsustained ventricular tachycardias, but it should not be used for this indication in patients who have underlying heart disease. This finding was made apparent by results of the Cardiac Arrhythmia Suppression Trial (CAST), which tested the proposition that suppression of ventricular ectopy after myocardial infarction would reduce mortality. Patients receiving flecainide or encainide in this trial had significantly higher mortality than did patients receiving placebo. The significant difference has been attributed to the proarrhytmic properties of the Class IC drugs.

Adverse Effects and Interactions: Flecainide is generally better tolerated than most antiarrhythmic agents. Mild to moderate visual disturbances are the most common side effect, usually manifesting as blurred vision. Occasionally gastrointestinal symptoms occur. However, no significant organ toxicity has been reported.

By far the most serious adverse effect of flecainide (and of all Class IC drugs) is its significant proarrhythmic potential (see the comparison to other Class I drugs in Table 3.7). Proarrhythmia with IC agents takes the form of exacerbation of reentrant ventricular tachycardia; torsades de pointes is not seen. Thus, proarrhythmia with flecainide is essentially limited to patients who have the potential for developing reentrant ventricular arrhythmias, that is, patients with underlying cardiac disease. CAST revealed that proarrhythmia with Class IC drugs is especially likely during times of acute myocardial ischemia. Perhaps ischemia magnifies the effect of these drugs as it does with both Class IA and IB drugs. In any case, flecainide and other Class IC drugs appear to have a tendency to convert an episode of angina to an episode of sudden death. Class IC drugs should be avoided in patients with coronary artery disease.

Flecainide levels may be increased by amiodarone, cimetidine, propranolol, and quinidine. Flecainide may modestly increase digoxin levels.

Encainide

Encainide is a Class IC drug whose electrophysiologic and clinical properties are very similar to those of flecainide. Encainide was removed from the market after CAST and is no longer available.

Propafenone

Propafenone was developed in the late 1960s and released for use in the United States in 1989.

Table 3.7. Common Adverse Effects of Class I Drugs

	General Toxicity	Proarrhythmia	
		Reentrant VT	Torsades
Quinidine	GI (diarrhea), cinchonism, rashes, hemolytic anemia, thrombocytopenia	++	++
Procainamide	Hypotension (IV), lupus, GI (nausea), agranulocytosis	++	++
Disopyramide	Cardiac decompensation, urinary retention, dry mouth and eyes	++	++
Lidocaine	CNS (slurred speech, paresthesias, seizures)	+	−
Mexiletine	GI (nausea), CNS (tremor, ataxia)	+	−
Phenytoin	GI (nausea), CNS (ataxia, nystagmus), hypersensitivity reactions (rashes, hematologic), osteomalacia, megaloblastic anemia	+	−
Flecainide	Visual disturbances, GI (nausea), cardiac decompensation	+++	−
Propafenone	GI (nausea), CNS (dizziness, ataxia), cardiac decompensation (uncommon)	+++	−
Moricizine	Dizziness, headache, nausea	++	−

Clinical Pharmacology: Propafenone is well absorbed from the gastrointestinal tract and achieves peak blood levels 2 to 3 hours after an oral dose. It is subject to extensive first-pass hepatic metabolism that results in nonlinear kinetics—as the dosage of the drug is increased, hepatic metabolism becomes saturated; thus, a relatively small increase in dosage can produce a relatively large increase in drug levels. The drug is 90% protein bound and is metabolized by the liver. The elimination half-life is 6 or 7 hours after a steady-state is reached. Generally, 3 days at a stable drug dosage achieves steady-state blood levels.

Dosage: The usual dosage of propafenone is 150–300 mg every 8 hours. Generally, the beginning dosage is 150 mg or 225 mg every 8 hours. Dosage may be increased, but not more often than every third day.

Electrophysiologic Effects: Propafenone produces potent blockade of the sodium channel, similar to other Class IC drugs. Unlike other Class IC agents, however, propafenone also causes a slight increase in the refractory periods of all cardiac tissue. In addition, propafenone has mild beta-blocking and calcium-blocking properties.

Hemodynamic Effects: Propafenone has a negative inotropic effect that is relatively mild, substantially less than that seen with disopyramide or flecainide. The drug also blunts the heart rate during exercise. Both effects may be a result of its beta-blocking (and perhaps its calcium-blocking) properties.

Therapeutic Uses: Like all Class IC agents, propafenone is effective against a wide variety of atrial and ventricular arrhythmias. Its therapeutic profile is similar to that of flecainide.

Adverse Effects and Interactions: The most common side effects are dizziness, lightheadedness, ataxia, nausea, and a metallic aftertaste. Exacerbation of congestive heart failure can be seen, especially in patients with histories of heart failure. Generally, propafenone tends to cause more nonproarrhythmic side effects than do other Class IC antiarrhythmic drugs.

As is the case with all Class IC drugs, proarrhythmia is a significant problem with propafenone, but the problem is limited to patients with underlying heart disease. Most clinicians believe that proarrhythmia with propafenone is somewhat less frequent than it is with flecainide.

Numerous drug interactions have been reported with propafenone. Phenobarbital, phenytoin, and rifampin decrease levels of propafenone. Quinidine and cimetidine increase levels of propafenone. Propafenone increases levels of digoxin, propranolol, metoprolol, theophylline, cyclosporine, and desipramine. It increases the effect of warfarin.

Moricizine

Moricizine, a phenothiazine derivative, has been in use in Russia since the 1970s. It was approved by the FDA in 1990.

Clinical Pharmacology: Moricizine is absorbed almost completely when administered orally, and peak plasma levels occur within 1 to 2 hours. Moricizine is extensively metabolized in the liver to a multitude of compounds, some of which may have electrophysiologic effects. The elimination half-life of the parent compound is variable (generally 3 to 12 hr), but the half-life of some of its metabolites is substantially longer. Plasma levels of moricizine have not reflected efficacy of the drug.

Dosage: Moricizine is usually initiated in dosages of 200 mg orally every 8 hours and may be increased to 250–300 mg every 8 hours. Generally, it is recommended that dosage increases be made no more often than every third day. Dosage should be decreased in the presence of hepatic insufficiency.

Electrophysiologic Effects: Moricizine does not display the same affinity for the sodium channel displayed by other Class IC drugs. Hence, its effect on conduction velocity is less pronounced than that for flecainide or propafenone. In addition, moricizine decreases the action potential duration and therefore decreases refractory periods, similar to Class IB agents. Classification of moricizine has thus been controversial—some classify it as an IB drug. It is classified as an IC drug in this chapter mainly to emphasize its proarrhythmic effects (which are only rarely seen with Class IB drugs).

Hemodynamic Effects: Moricizine may have a mild negative inotropic effect, but in general, exacerbation of congestive heart failure has been uncommon with this drug.

Therapeutic Uses: Moricizine is moderately effective in the treatment of both atrial and ventricular arrhythmias. It has been used successfully in treating bypass-tract-mediated tachyarrhythmias and may have some efficacy against atrial fibrillation and atrial flutter. Its efficacy against ventricular arrhythmias is generally greater than that of Class IB agents but is clearly less than that for other Class IC drugs. A tendency for higher mortality with moricizine compared with that for placebo was seen in CAST, but the study was terminated before the tendency reached statistical significance.

Adverse Effects and Interactions: In general, moricizine is fairly well tolerated. Most side effects are related to the gastrointestinal or central nervous systems, similar to Class IB drugs. Dizziness, headache, and nausea are the most common side effects.

Proarrhythmia clearly occurs with moricizine more often than it does with Class IB drugs but less often than that with other Class IC drugs.

Cimetidine increases moricizine levels and moricizine decreases theophylline levels.

Class II Antiarrhythmic Drugs: Beta-Blocking Agents

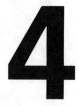

Beta-blocking drugs exert antiarrhythmic effects by blunting the arrhythmogenic actions of catecholamines. Compared with other antiarrhythmic drugs, these agents are only mediocre at suppressing overt cardiac arrhythmias. Nonetheless, beta blockers exert a powerful protective effect in certain clinical conditions—they are among the few drugs that have been shown to significantly reduce the incidence of sudden death in any subset of patients (an effect they most likely achieve by preventing cardiac arrhythmias).

Because of the success of the drugs in treating a myriad of medical problems, more than two dozen beta blockers have been synthesized, and more than a dozen are available for clinical use in the United States. In contrast to Class I antiarrhythmic drugs, the antiarrhythmic effects of Class II drugs tend to be quite similar to one another.

ELECTROPHYSIOLOGIC EFFECTS OF BETA BLOCKERS

For practical purposes, the electrophysiologic effects of beta blockers are manifested solely by their blunting of the actions of catecholamines. The effect of beta blockers on the cardiac electrical system, then, reflects the distribution of adrenergic innervation of the heart. In areas in which there is rich adrenergic innervation, beta blockers can have a pronounced effect. In areas in which adrenergic innervation is sparse, the electrophysiologic effect of beta blockers is relatively minimal.

Since adrenergic stimulation is most pronounced in the sinoatrial (SA) and atrioventricular (AV) nodes, it is in these structures that beta blockers have their greatest electrophysiologic effects. In both the SA and AV nodes, phase 4 depolarization is blunted by beta-blocking agents, leading to a decrease in automaticity, and hence a slowing in the heart rate. In the AV node, beta blockers cause a marked slowing in conduction and a prolongation in refractory periods. The drugs have relatively little effect on SA nodal conduction in normal individuals, but can markedly prolong SA nodal conduction (leading to sinus nodal exit block and hence bradyarrhythmias) in patients with intrinsic SA nodal disease. Beta blockers have very little effect on conduction velocity or refractoriness in normal atrial or ventricular myocardium.

Beta blockers can have a profound electrophysiologic effect, however, in ischemic or damaged myocardium. By helping to prevent ischemia, the drugs can reduce the incidence of arrhythmias. Further, beta blockers raise the threshold for ventricular fibrillation in ischemic myocardium and have been shown to reduce the risk of ventricular fibrillation during ischemia. There is also evidence that beta blockers can help prevent the formation of reentrant arrhythmias in myocardium that has been damaged by ischemia. In such damaged myocardium, a maldistribution of autonomic innervation can arise and lead to regional differences in adrenergic stimulation. Regional differences can serve as substrate for reentrant tachyarrhythmias by creating localized differences in refractory periods. By smoothing out localized differences in autonomic stimulation, beta blockers can prevent arrhythmias.

BETA-BLOCKING AGENTS IN THE TREATMENT OF ARRHYTHMIAS
Supraventricular Arrhythmias

The major effects of beta blockers are manifested in the SA and AV nodes; it should not be surprising that the efficacy of beta blockers in treating supraventricular arrhythmias is mainly related to the extent to which the arrhythmias depend on the SA and AV nodes. Beta blockers tend to be most effective for supraventricular arrhythmias in which the SA or AV nodes are included within the reentrant pathways (SA nodal reentrant tachycardia, AV nodal reentrant tachycardia, and macroreentrant tachycardias associated with bypass tracts). In these arrhythmias beta blockers can have a direct suppressive effect on the pathways of reentry thus, they can

Table 4.1.   Potential Effects of Beta-Blocking Drugs on Supraventricular Tachyarrhythmias

Terminate or Prevent
  AV nodal reentrant tachycardia
  SA nodal reentrant tachycardia
  Macroreentrant (bypass-tract-mediated) tachycardia
Slow Ventricular Response
  Atrial tachycardia (automatic or reentrant)
  Atrial fibrillation
  Atrial flutter

terminate the arrhythmias themselves, and can help prevent the onset of recurrent arrhythmias.

For arrhythmias arising within the atrial muscle (automatic or reentrant atrial tachycardias, atrial fibrillation, and atrial flutter), beta blockers tend to have minimal direct suppressive effect. In these atrial arrhythmias, however, beta blockers can still be quite useful in helping to control the ventricular response by increasing the refractory period of the AV node and thus allowing fewer impulses to be transmitted to the ventricles. In rare patients, beta blockers also help to prevent arrhythmias arising in the atria. In such patients, atrial arrhythmias appear to be catechol dependent; patients often relate the onset of their arrhythmias to exercise. The effects of beta blockers are summarized in Table 4.1.

Ventricular Arrhythmias

In general, beta blockers are not particularly effective at suppressing ambient ventricular ectopy or ventricular tachycardias. In some circumstances, however, generally when arrhythmias are related to catecholamines or to myocardial ischemia, beta blockers can be useful. Beta blockers are the drugs of choice, for instance, for exercise-induced ventricular arrhythmias. Beta blockers also have been shown to reduce the number of episodes of ventricular fibrillation during acute myocardial infarction, significantly improve overall survival, and reduce the risk of sudden death and recurrent infarction in survivors of myocardial infarction.

Beta blockers can also be effective in treating the long QT interval syndrome. This condition, usually congenital, is characterized by a long QT interval and a propensity for syncope or sudden death during exercise or during times of severe emotional stress.

There is no consensus on the mechanism of the ventricular tachyarrhythmias that produce these events. The most likely mechanisms are delayed afterdepolarizations (DADs) or localized differences in refractory periods caused by a maldistribution of sympathetic fibers in the ventricles. In the latter, beta blockers (which along with left stellate sympathectomy have been effective in treating many patients with this disorder) might be expected to smooth out any resultant sympathetic imbalance and render less likely arrhythmias mediated by nonuniform refractory periods.

CLINICAL PHARMACOLOGY OF BETA-BLOCKING AGENTS

To a large extent, all the marketed beta blockers appear to be of comparable efficacy in the treatment of arrhythmias and ischemia. Choosing among these agents, then, is mainly a matter of selecting a drug with an appropriate pharmacologic profile for the patient being treated. Among the considerations in making such a selection are the relative potencies of the drugs being considered and whether they offer receptor selectivity, intrinsic sympathomimetic activity (ISA), vasodilator activity, and membrane-stabilizing activity. Table 4.2 is not all inclusive, but it lists the pharmacologic properties of the most commonly used beta-blocking agents.

Potency of a beta blocker is not a major consideration, but the recommended dosages of various beta blockers differ markedly, and dosages must be adjusted accordingly for the drug being used.

Table 4.2. Clinical Pharmacology of Beta-Blocking Drugs

Drug	β_1-Selective	ISA	Class I	Vasodilator	Lipid-Soluble	Half-Life (hr)
Acebutolol	+	+	+	0	Moderate	3–10
Atenolol	++	0	0	0	Weak	6–9
Carvedilol	0	0	++	+	Moderate	7–10
Esmolol	++	0	0	+	Weak	9 min
Labetolol	0	+	0	+	Weak	3–4
Metoprolol	++	0	0	0	Moderate	3–4
Pindolol	0	++	+	0	Moderate	3–4
Propranolol	0	0	++	0	High	3–4
Timolol	0	0	0	0	Weak	4–5

ISA = intrinsic sympathomimetic activity.

Receptor selectivity refers to β_1-receptors (those in the heart) and β_2-receptors (those in the peripheral vasculature and bronchi). Drugs with selectivity, such as atenolol and metoprolol, produce minimal blockade of β_2-receptors, and are thus potentially safer to use in patients with lung disease or with impaired peripheral circulation.

ISA refers to the fact that some beta blockers, such as pindolol and acebutolol, produce a partial agonist (stimulating) effect on the beta receptor sites to which they bind (and block). Thus, in theory, heart rate depression and depression of myocardial function might not be as potent with beta blockers offering ISA. However, clear-cut clinical indications for using ISA drugs have not been identified. Of note, drugs offering ISA may not have a protective effect in survivors of myocardial infarction.

Vasodilator activity is produced by some beta blockers either through α_1-receptor blockade (carvedilol), or direct β_2-receptor stimulation (dilevalol), or both (labetolol).

Membrane-stabilizing activity refers to the fact that a few beta blockers exhibit Class I antiarrhythmic activity (slowing of the depolarization phase of the action potential) if serum levels are sufficiently high. However, the levels that must be achieved to demonstrate such Class I activity is greatly in excess of therapeutic levels. Thus, whether membrane-stabilizing activity is ever relevant with the use of beta blockers is very questionable.

The lipid solubility of beta blockers partially determines how the agents are metabolized (lipid-soluble drugs are generally metabolized in the liver and water-soluble drugs are generally excreted by the kidneys) and whether they cross the blood-brain barrier (drugs that cross are more prone to cause central nervous system side effects such as fatigue, depression, insomnia, or hallucinations).

In summary, beta blockers as a class generally exhibit similar efficacies in the treatment of cardiac arrhythmias. The major considerations in choosing among these drugs are the predominant route of elimination (to avoid accumulation of the drug in a patient with liver or kidney disease), side effects, and whether receptor selectivity or vasodilation are desired. In general, the potential for membrane-stabilizing activity should be ignored and ISA avoided.

ADVERSE EFFECTS AND DRUG INTERACTIONS

The most common side effects of beta blockers are a direct consequence of adrenergic blockade—bradyarrhythmias, myocardial depression, bronchoconstriction, claudication, Raynaud's phenomenon, intensification of hypoglycemic episodes, fatigue, sexual dysfunction, mental depression, and nightmares. Other side effects are rashes, fever, and gastrointestinal symptoms. In diabetics, beta blockers can mask symptoms of hypoglycemia and can cause hypoglycemia by reducing gluconeogenesis or hyperglycemia by reducing insulin levels.

Some side effects related to beta blockade itself may be avoided by appropriate drug selection. As noted, drugs with β_1-selectivity might help in avoiding bronchospasm, worsening of hypoglycemia, claudication, and Raynaud's phenomenon in some individuals. Using drugs with low lipid solubility might help to prevent central nervous system side effects.

Hepatic metabolism of lipid-soluble beta blockers can be increased by cimetidine and decreased by barbiturates. Aluminum hydroxide can delay absorbtion of beta blockers. The hepatic metabolism of lidocaine can be reduced by administration of lipophilic beta blockers such as propranolol.

Class III Antiarrhythmic Drugs

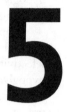

Class III antiarrhythmic drugs prolong the duration of the cardiac action potential, usually by blocking the potassium channels that mediate repolarization, and thus increase the refractory periods of cardiac tissue (Figure 5.1).

Despite this defining similarity, none of the currently available Class III drugs behave exactly alike. One reason the drugs are clinically dissimilar is that none are pure Class III agents—all have additional electrophysiologic effects that contribute to their efficacy and to their toxicity. Another reason for differences among the Class III drugs is that they display varying degrees of reverse use dependence.

The term *use dependence* refers to the time-related effect of Class I drugs on the sodium channel; as a result of binding kinetics, the effect of the drugs on sodium blockade increases as the heart rate increases. The magnitude of potassium-channel blockade manifested by Class III agents, it turns out, also is related to heart rate. In this case, however, the strength of blockade *decreases* as the heart rate increases; hence, the term *reverse use dependence*. Reverse use dependence means that at slow heart rates the prolongation of the action potential is most pronounced; at faster heart rates the effect diminishes. Reverse use dependence is related to a drug's binding characteristics. Drugs that preferentially bind to closed potassium channels, for instance, display significant reverse use dependence because phase 4 of the action potential is longer (and thus potassium channels spend more time in the closed state) when the heart rate is slow. Reverse use dependence has two potential undesirable effects. First, this property causes some Class III drugs to lose potency with rapid heart rates just when one would want

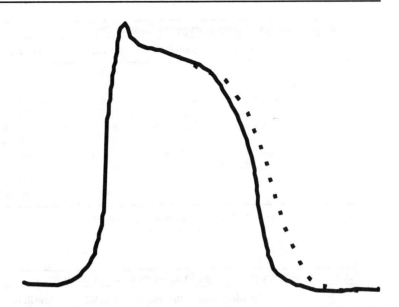
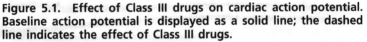

Figure 5.1. Effect of Class III drugs on cardiac action potential. Baseline action potential is displayed as a solid line; the dashed line indicates the effect of Class III drugs.

the drugs to be most effective. Second, the fact that action potential prolongation by some Class III drugs is most pronounced during bradycardia potentiates the tendency to cause torsades de pointes, an arrhythmia that is most likely to occur after pauses.

Amiodarone is unusual for a Class III agent in that it binds preferentially to open potassium channels and therefore displays much less reverse use dependence. Consequently, amiodarone does not lose much of its effect when heart rate increases. The low magnitude of reverse use dependence seen with amiodarone may explain not only its remarkable efficacy against tachyarrhythmias but also its low incidence of producing torsades de pointes.

Although the differences among Class III drugs have not yet mandated that this class be subgrouped as the Class I drugs have been, the rush to develop new Class III drugs will almost certainly eventually lead to such a subgrouping. For now, it is sufficient to keep in mind that these drugs are not interchangeable. The major clinical features of Class III antiarrhythmic drugs are listed in Table 5.1, and the major electrophysiologic properties are listed in Table 5.2.

Table 5.1. Clinical Pharmacology of Class III Drugs

	Amiodarone	Bretylium	Sotalol	Ibutilide
GI absorption	30–50%	—	>90%	—
Elimination	Hepatic*	Renal	Renal	Renal
Half-life	30–106 days	9–10 hr	12 hr	2–12 hr
Dosage range	800–1600 mg/day for 3–10 days, then 100–400 mg/day PO	5 mg/kg IV, 1–2 mg/min IV infusion	160–320 mg/day PO	10-mg IV infusion during 10 min, may be repeated

* Both hepatic and renal elimination are minimal for amiodarone.
GI = gastrointestinal; IV = intravenous; PO = oral.

Table 5.2. Electrophysiologic Properties of Class III Drugs

	Amiodarone	Bretylium	Sotalol	Ibutilide
Conduction velocity	Decrease +	0	0	0
Refractory periods	Increase++	Increase++	Increase++	Increase++
Automaticity	Suppress++	Suppress+	Suppress+	Suppress+
Afterdepolarizations	May cause EADs	May cause EADs	May cause EADs	May cause EADs
Other effects	Class II and Class IV	Antiadren-ergic	Class II	
Efficacy				
Atrial fib/flutter	++	0	++	++
AVN reentry	+++	0	++	0
Macroreentry	+++	0	++	0
PVCs	+++	+	++	0
VT/VF	+++	+++	++	0

AVN = AV node; EADs = early afterdepolarizations; PVCs = premature ventricular complexes; VT/VF = ventricular tachycardia and ventricular fibrillation.

AMIODARONE

Amiodarone was synthesized in Belgium in the 1960s as a vasodilator. Its antiarrhythmic efficacy was noted in the early 1970s, and the drug quickly came into use in many countries as an antiarrhythmic agent. In the late 1970s, clinical trials with amiodarone were begun in the United States and the oral form of the drug was approved by the Food and Drug Administration (FDA) in the mid-1980s. The intravenous form was approved in 1995.

Electrophysiologic Effects

Amiodarone displays activity from all four antiarrhythmic classes. It is classified as a Class III antiarrhythmic drug because its major electrophysiologic effect is a homogeneous prolongation of the action potential, and therefore of refractoriness, in all cardiac tissues. Prolongation of refractoriness is not seen immediately. It gradually increases throughout the period of amiodarone loading and may not become maximal for several weeks. Little change in refractoriness is seen acutely with intravenous loading of the drug.

In addition to its potassium-channel effects, amiodarone produces a mild to moderate blockade of the sodium channel (a Class I effect), a noncompetitive beta blockade (a Class II effect), and some degree of calcium-channel blockade (a Class IV effect). All the effects can produce antiarrhythmic actions.

Clinical Pharmacology

The clinical pharmacology of amiodarone can fairly be described as being bizarre, complex, and incompletely understood. After an oral dose, 30% to 50% is absorbed from the gastrointestinal tract. Once absorbed, amiodarone displays a complex pattern of distribution that is usually described as (at least) a three-compartment model. The first, or central, compartment is thought to consist of the intravascular space. With aggressive loading regimens, the central compartment can be largely saturated within 24 hours. The second, or peripheral, compartment probably consists of most of the body's organs. It is thought to take 5 to 7 days to begin to saturate the peripheral compartment by use of a typical regimen for loading amiodarone—an important consideration because the antiarrhythmic effects of amiodarone are thought to require adequate filling of the peripheral compartment. The third, or deep, compartment consists of the body's fat. It takes many weeks or months for the third compartment to become saturated. Because of the depth of the deep compartment, amiodarone has a huge volume of distribution; it has been calculated to be as high as 500 liters. Tissue concentrations of amiodarone vary markedly from organ to organ and are the highest in organs with high fat content, such as the liver and the lungs. In vivo, amiodarone is in a state of equilibrium among the three compartments. If the drug is discontinued, the concentration of amiodarone in the central compartment (the serum) falls quickly to low levels, but the low serum levels persist for weeks or months because of the slow leaching of the drug from the peripheral and deep compartments.

Amiodarone is metabolized in the liver to desethylamiodarone (DEA), which displays electrophysiologic effects similar to the parent compound and has similar pharmacologic properties. Very little amiodarone or DEA is excreted in the urine or the stool; essentially, amiodarone is stored, not excreted. The half-life of the drug has been reported as 2 weeks to 3 months in duration. The very long half-life is reflected in the low daily dosage requirement after loading has been achieved.

Dosage

The unusual kinetics of amiodarone dictate the loading schedule. Usually, 1200–1600 mg/day are given in divided doses for several days (usually 5 to 14 days), followed by 400–600 mg/day for several weeks, and finally by a chronic maintenance dose of 200–400 mg/ day. This sort of loading regimen has been arrived at empirically, but it is a logical approach. By giving large doses for days to weeks, one can achieve relatively rapid saturation of the central and peripheral compartments. Achieving a steady state, however, requires filling the deep compartment, which takes many weeks.

When treating non–life-threatening arrhythmias or when using amiodarone as prophylaxis against arrhythmias that are not manifest, a much milder loading regimen is often used. Less aggressive loading schedules may avoid some toxicities associated with administering higher doses of the drug but require significantly more time to achieve both an antiarrhythmic effect and a steady state.

Recently, the intravenous form of amiodarone has been approved in the United States, and there has already been confusion regarding its appropriate use. Intravenous amiodarone should not be thought of as creating new indications for the drug. Instead, it should be thought of merely as an alternative method of administering the drug when the decision has been made to load a patient with amiodarone. Specifically, intravenous amiodarone has not been demonstrated to have a more rapid onset of action than that of rapid oral loading. The Class III effects of amiodarone are not seen acutely with IV loading—relatively long-term administration of the drug is necessary before prolongation of refractoriness is seen, just as with oral loading. The immediate effects of intrave-

Table 5.3. Electrophysiologic Effects of IV Versus PO Amiodarone*

Administration	QT Interval	AH Interval	Atrial RP	Ventricular RP
PO	Increase	Increase	Increase	Increase
IV	—	Increase	—	—

*The AH interval reflects the refractory period of the AV node. PO administration of amiodarone (after sufficient loading) results in prolongation of the action potential, as reflected by the resultant increase in the QT interval and in atrial and ventricular refractory periods; acute IV loading does not. The Class III effects of amiodarone are not seen with acute IV loading; instead, the increase in AV nodal refractoriness indicates that the Class II (and possibly Class IV) effects of amiodarone predominate.
RP = refractory periods.

nous amiodarone are limited mainly to its Class II (beta-blocking) actions (Table 5.3). Accordingly, the most prominent electrophysiologic effect is prolongation of the atrioventricular (AV) nodal refractory periods, and the most prominent hemodynamic effect is hypotension. Any immediate antiarrhythmic efficacy with intravenous amiodarone is likely to be at least partially related to how dependent a patient's arrhythmias are on catecholamine stimulation.

When amiodarone is loaded intravenously, 1 g is delivered during the first 24 hours as follows: 150 mg is infused during the first 10 minutes (15 mg/min), followed by 360 mg during the next 6 hours (1 mg/min), and then followed by 540 mg during the next 18 hours (0.5 mg/min). If intravenous therapy is still desired after the first 24 hours, the infusion can continue at 0.5 mg/min (720 mg/24 hr). Note that the intravenous regimen may not be more rapid (and possibly no more efficacious) than that of many aggressive oral loading regimens.

Indications

Amiodarone is a broad spectrum antiarrhythmic agent. It can be efficacious for virtually any type of tachyarrhythmia.

Amiodarone is moderately effective in maintaining sinus rhythm in patients with atrial tachyarrhythmias, including atrial fibrillation and atrial flutter. It is often effective in bypass-tract-mediated tachycardias and works moderately well for AV nodal reentrant tachycardias.

Amiodarone is the most effective drug ever developed for the treatment of ventricular tachycardia and ventricular fibrillation.

Early studies with amiodarone generally limited its use to patients whose ventricular tachyarrhythmias had proven refractory (most often, as documented during electrophysiologic testing) to other antiarrhythmic therapy. Even in this difficult-to-treat population, amiodarone has reduced the risk of sudden death to about half that seen with more conventional drugs.

Amiodarone's use as a prophylactic agent for survivors of myocardial infarction or for patients with congestive heart failure has been the subject of several randomized trials but remains controversial. The prophylactic use of amiodarone is discussed in more detail in Chapter 11.

Adverse Effects and Interactions

Amiodarone causes a high incidence of side effects ranging from merely annoying to life-threatening. Many side effects of amiodarone appear to be related to the total lifetime cumulative dose of the drug (rather than to the daily dosage), so the risk of developing new side effects continues to increase as therapy continues over time.

Gastrointestinal side effects are common but tend to be mild. Nausea, vomiting, or anorexia have an incidence of approximately 25% during the high-dose loading phase, but these symptoms often improve with lowering of the daily dosage. Elevation of liver function tests is not uncommon. The consequences of chronically elevated hepatic transaminases caused by amiodarone are unclear, although some cases of amiodarone-induced hepatitis have been reported. Esophageal reflux caused by an amiodarone-induced paralysis of the lower esophageal sphincter is an uncommon but potentially devastating side effect.

Pulmonary complications are generally considered the most dangerous side effect seen with amiodarone. Acute adult respiratory distress syndrome from amiodarone-induced pneumonitis can be seen at any time during therapy, but the time of highest risk for the condition is probably immediately after surgery, especially cardiac surgery. The incidence of acute amiodarone-induced pneumonitis is generally reported to be 2% to 5%, but the cumulative incidence is probably higher with long-term therapy. A chronic interstitial fibrosis also can be seen with amiodarone; the incidence of this problem is unclear. The carbon monoxide (CO) diffusing capacity is almost always depressed with amiodarone-induced pulmonary problems, but this laboratory finding is unfortunately nonspecific—

many patients taking amiodarone develop depressed CO diffusing capacities without clinically apparent pulmonary problems.

Thyroid problems with amiodarone are relatively common. Amiodarone reduces peripheral conversion of T_4 to T_3, resulting in somewhat increased T_4 levels and somewhat decreased T_3 levels even in euthyroid patients. Approximately 10% of patients treated with amiodarone eventually develop true hypothyroidism (a low serum T_4 level is always significant in patients taking this drug), and a smaller proportion develop hyperthyroidism. Although hypothyroidism can be treated easily with thyroid replacement medication, hyperthyroidism represents a difficult clinical problem because of its presentation and its treatment. Amiodarone-induced hyperthyroidism sometimes manifests as an exacerbation of the patient's underlying ventricular tachyarrhythmias. This is a potentially lethal condition. Further, because amiodarone itself contains a significant amount of iodine, patients receiving amiodarone have high iodine stores, which thus precludes the use of radioactive iodine for thyroid ablation. To make matters worse, treating amiodarone-induced hyperthyroidism with antithyroid drugs is always difficult and often impossible. Frequently, thyroidectomy is the only feasible means of controlling amiodarone-induced hyperthyroidism.

Cutaneous side effects with amiodarone are relatively frequent. Significant photosensitivity occurs in about 20% of patients taking the drug, and some patients eventually develop a blue-gray discoloration of sun-exposed skin, which can be quite disfiguring.

Neurologic side effects are rare but can include ataxia, tremor, sleep disturbances, and peripheral neuropathy. A proximal myopathy can also be seen with amiodarone.

Ocular symptoms (most often, poor night vision) occasionally accompany the corneal microdeposits seen in virtually all patients taking amiodarone.

Multiple drug interactions have been reported with amiodarone. The most common are the potentiation of warfarin and increased digoxin levels. Quinidine, procainamide, phenytoin, and flecainide levels are also increased. As a rule, if amiodarone is given in combination with Class I antiarrhythmic drugs, the dosage of the Class I drug should be decreased. Amiodarone can potentiate the effect of beta blockers and calcium blockers and lead to negative inotropic effects and bradyarrhythmias.

BRETYLIUM

Breytlium was developed in the 1950s as an antihypertensive agent, but because of its poor oral absorption, it was never marketed for this indication. Its antiarrhythmic properties were noted in the 1960s.

Electrophysiologic Effects

Bretylium displays Class III antiarrhythmic behavior—it causes prolongation in the duration of the action potential in ventricular myocardium. Bretylium is taken up by the peripheral adrenergic nerve terminals and ultimately blocks release and reuptake of norepinephrine, which produces an antiadrenergic effect. Initially, however, bretylium causes release of norepinephrine from the nerve terminal and leads to an initial adrenergic surge whose magnitude is quite variable from patient to patient.

Bretylium also displays an antifibrillatory action, but whether this is caused by its Class III effects, its antiadrenergic effects, or some other mechanism (the drug, for instance, also alters prostaglandin levels) is unclear. The drug also appears to lower the energy level required to defibrillate the ventricles.

Clinical Pharmacology

Bretylium is limited to intravenous use because it is poorly absorbed from the gut. The drug is extensively tissue bound; after several hours, the myocardial concentration of the drug can be 10 times higher than the serum concentration. Bretylium is excreted by the kidneys, but because of its tissue binding, the elimination half-life is relatively long—9 or 10 hours.

Dosage

Bretylium is given intravenously as an initial bolus of 5 mg/kg during a period of 10 minutes, followed by an infusion of 1–2 mg/min. The bolus can be repeated after 30 minutes.

Indications

The use of bretylium is limited to emergency situations to prevent recurrent ventricular fibrillation.

Adverse Effects

The most common side effects of bretylium are hypotension (which is largely postural in nature) and symptoms relating to the initial adrenergic surge caused by the drug (which include tachycardia, hypertension, flushing, and the production of ventricular arrhythmias). The latter symptoms usually last only a few minutes but can sometimes persist longer than 1 hour. Nausea and vomiting can also occur after administration of bretylium. Bretylium does not appear to cause torsades de pointes; any proarrhythmic potential appears to be a result of the initial adrenergic surge.

SOTALOL

Sotalol, a noncardioselective beta blocker, was initially developed as an antihypertensive agent. Its Class III antiarrhythmic properties were noted in 1970, and it began to be studied as an antiarrhythmic agent at that time.

Electrophysiologic Properties

Sotalol is a Class III antiarrhythmic drug; it produces prolongation of the cardiac action potential in both the atria and the ventricles. It produces a dose-related prolongation in the QT interval, which appears to reflect both its antiarrhythmic properties and its propensity to cause torsades de pointes. The marketed compound is actually a racemic mixture of D-sotalol (which has Class III effects), and L-sotalol (which has beta-blocking effects). As a beta blocker, sotalol is about one-third as potent as propranolol.

Clinical Pharmacology

Sotalol is well absorbed from the gastrointestinal tract, and peak plasma concentrations occur within 2 to 3 hours after an oral dose. The drug is not metabolized; it is excreted unchanged by the kidneys. The elimination half-life is 7 to 8 hours.

Dosage

The usual starting dosage of sotalol is 80 mg twice daily, and the dosage is increased gradually, as needed, to 240–320 mg/day in divided doses. Intervals of at least 2 or 3 days between dosage increments are recommended. Careful monitoring of the QT interval must be performed while titrating the dose because the risk of developing torsades de pointes with sotalol is clearly related to QT prolongation. The corrected QT interval should be kept below 500 milliseconds to keep the risk of torsades under 2%. Dosage greater than 320 mg/day may be necessary to suppress arrhythmias, but higher doses lead to a substantial increase in the incidence of torsades de pointes (as high as 11% in patients whose corrected QT interval exceeds 550 msec).

Indications

Sotalol is approved for the treatment of significant ventricular arrhythmias but can be useful for treating all types of tachyarrhythmias. The drug is generally considered more effective than Class IA drugs but not as effective as amiodarone.

Adverse Effects and Drug Interactions

The major side effects of sotalol are related to its noncardioselective beta-blocking effects (e.g., bradyarrhythmias, negative inotropy, exacerbation of asthma) and to its propensity to cause torsades. Exacerbation of congestive heart failure is most commonly seen in patients whose left ventricular ejection fractions are less than 0.35, especially if the patients also have a history of heart failure.

Torsades de pointes is of more concern with sotalol than it is with Class IA drugs or with amiodarone. As noted, the risk of torsades with sotalol (as opposed to any other drug yet available) is directly related to the magnitude of its Class III effects, as reflected by the duration of the QT interval. The higher the dose and the longer the QT interval, the higher the risk. Because sotalol displays reverse use dependence, its effect on the QT interval is even more profound at slower heart rates. So, for instance, if sotalol is being used to treat atrial fibrillation, the relative safety of using the drug (i.e., the magnitude of QT interval prolongation) *must* be assessed during sinus rhythm, that is, when the heart rate is slowest and the risk of torsades is highest. Thus, such a patient should never be sent home taking sotalol until the person has been observed in sinus rhythm. Hypokalemia also magnifies the incidence of sotalol-induced torsades. Therefore, the drug should be used with trepidation in patients taking potassium-wasting diuretics—another good reason to avoid the drug in patients with congestive heart failure. Recently, a multicenter randomized trial using D-sotalol in patients with ventricular arrhythmias was stopped because of an excess of sudden death in the D-sotalol arm. Presumably, torsades was largely responsible for the excess mortality.

Concomitant use of Class IA drugs can greatly magnify the risk of torsades. Sotalol can potentiate, in an additive fashion, the negative inotropic and bradyarrhythmic effects of other beta-blocking agents and of calcium-blocking drugs.

IBUTILIDE

Ibutilide is a new Class III antiarrhythmic agent recently approved by the FDA in its intravenous form for the acute cardioversion of atrial fibrillation and atrial flutter.

Electrophysiologic Properties

Ibutilide is a unique Class III drug in that it causes prolongation of the action potential by blocking inward sodium currents rather than outward potassium currents. Like sotalol, the drug produces a dose-related prolongation in the QT interval.

Clinical Pharmacology

After intravenous infusion, ibutilide is extensively metabolized to eight metabolites. More than 80% of the drug is excreted in the urine, only 7% as unmetabolized ibutilide. The elimination half-life is variable (2 to 12 hr) but averages 6 hours.

Dosage

Ibutilide is infused as a 1-mg intravenous bolus during a period of 10 minutes. If the arrhythmia being treated (atrial fibrillation or atrial flutter) persists for 10 minutes after the infusion has been completed, a second 1-mg bolus can be administered. The infusion should be stopped immediately if the target arrhythmia is terminated or if ventricular arrhythmias or a marked prolongation of the QT interval are seen. After the infusion has been completed, the patient should be observed on a cardiac monitor for at least 4 hours or until the QT interval returns to normal, whichever is longer.

Indications

Ibutilide is indicated for the elective conversion of atrial fibrillation or atrial flutter. It should be thought of as an alternative to elective direct current (DC) cardioversion. In clinical studies, the efficacy of ibutilide administration in terminating these arrhythmias (after two 1-mg doses) was 44%.

Adverse Effects and Drug Interactions

The major adverse effect of ibutilide is its propensity to cause torsades de pointes. During clinical trials, ibutilide was not given to patients whose corrected QT intervals were greater than 440 milliseconds, and serum potassium levels were required to be greater than 4.0 mEq/liter. Despite these precautions, ventricular tachyarrhythmias were seen in some patients. Sustained ventricular arrhythmias requiring emergent cardioversion were seen in 1.7%, and nonsustained ventricular tachycardias were seen in 4.9%. The incidence of sustained ventricular arrhythmias was much higher in patients with a history of congestive heart failure (5.4%). Most ventricular arrhythmias were seen within 1 hour of the drug infusion, but some were seen approximately 3 hours after the infusion. More recently, a series was reported in which the incidence of ventricular arrhythmias after infusion of ibutilide was nearly 10%.

It is thought that the arrhythmogenic potential of ibutilide is increased when it is used with other drugs that prolong the duration of the action potential. Thus, ibutilide should not be used with Class IA or other Class III antiarrhythmic drugs, nor should these drugs be administered within 4 to 6 hours after infusion of ibutilide. Ibutilide should also be avoided in patients receiving phenothiazines, tricyclic antidepressants, tetracyclic antidepressants, or antihistamine agents that block the H_1 receptor.

Clinical Utility of Ibutilide

The overall clinical utility of ibutilide remains to be determined because of the disadvantages of the drug. Since only 44% of patients are effectively treated with ibutilide, more than half the patients treated with the drug require DC cardioversion. The incidence of torsades de pointes with ibutilide is also very troubling, and the relatively prolonged monitoring required after its use (regardless of whether it is effective) can be quite inconvenient. Overall, DC cardioversion should probably be used for most patients who require conversion from atrial fibrillation or atrial flutter.

Class IV Drugs:
Calcium-Blocking Agents

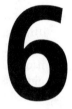

Of the many calcium-blocking agents that have been developed, only two are commonly used (and have been approved) for the treatment of cardiac arrhythmias: verapamil and diltiazem. For many other calcium-blocking agents, such as nifedipine, vasodilatory effects predominate; for these agents, reflex responses to vasodilation appear to counteract and cancel any cardiac electrophysiologic effects. Therefore, this chapter is limited to a discussion of verapamil and diltiazem.

CLINICAL PHARMACOLOGY OF VERAPAMIL AND DILTIAZEM

More than 90% of verapamil is absorbed after an oral dose, but first-pass hepatic metabolism reduces bioavailability to 20% to 35%. Approximately 90% of the drug is protein bound. With chronic administration, the elimination half-life is 5 to 12 hours. Very little verapamil is excreted unchanged in the urine. Verapamil can be given as an intravenous bolus for the emergent termination of reentrant supraventricular arrhythmias.

Diltiazem, like verapamil, is well absorbed but is subject to first-pass metabolism, yielding a bioavailability of about 40%. Diltiazem is 70% to 80% protein bound. The drug is metabolized in the liver, and the elimination half-life is approximately 3.5 hours. Diltiazem is also available for intravenous infusion, and is generally used in this form to control heart rate during atrial fibrillation or atrial flutter.

Dosage

The usual dosage of verapamil is 240–360 mg/day in divided doses given every 8 hours. Diltiazem is given four times a day, with a usual dosage range of 180–360 mg/day. Both drugs are now available in long-acting forms that can be given once or twice a day.

Verapamil can be given intravenously as a bolus. Five to 10 mg is administered during a period of 2 minutes; an additional 10 mg can be given after 10 minutes.

When giving diltiazem intravenously, 0.25 mg/kg (approximately 20–25 mg) should be given as a bolus during a period of 2 minutes, followed by infusion at 10 mg/hr. Infusion rates can be titrated to as much as 15 mg/hr depending on the response of the heart rate. The manufacturer does not recommend continuing diltiazem infusions for longer than 24 hours because longer infusion periods have not been studied.

Electrophysiologic Effects of Calcium-Blocking Agents

Calcium-blocking agents inhibit the slow calcium channel that is responsible for the depolarization of the sinoatrial (SA) and atrioventricular (AV) nodes. Accordingly, the major electrophysiologic effects of calcium-channel blockers are limited to these two structures. Both verapamil and diltiazem depress automaticity, slow conduction, and increase refractoriness in both the SA and AV nodes. The drugs are particularly useful in arrhythmias utilizing the AV node as part of the reentrant circuit.

As a general rule, calcium blockers have minimal or no electrophysiologic effect on the atrial or ventricular myocardium. However, the slow calcium channel has been invoked as a necessary component in the development of both early afterdepolarizations (EADs) and delayed afterdepolarizations (DADs). Calcium-channel blockers can occasionally ameliorate afterdepolarizations and the arrhythmias they cause. Further, it is apparent that the calcium channels might be responsible, on occasion, for localized areas of slow conduction in the ventricles. Thus, in relatively rare circumstances, calcium-channel blockers can be used to treat ventricular arrhythmias.

CLINICAL USE OF CALCIUM-BLOCKING AGENTS

Supraventricular Tachyarrhythmias

Verapamil and diltiazem can be very useful in the management of many supraventricular tachyarrhythmias either by affecting the mechanism of the arrhythmia itself and thus terminating or preventing the arrhythmia or in slowing the ventricular response to the arrhythmia.

Atrial Tachyarrhythmias: All these arrhythmias are localized to the atrial myocardium, so calcium blockers have very little direct effect on them. However, because calcium blockers increase the refractory period of the AV node, they can be very helpful in controlling the ventricular response during atrial tachyarrhythmias.

In general, it is easier to control ventricular response during atrial fibrillation than it is during atrial flutter or atrial tachycardia. With the latter two arrhythmias, changes in the ventricular rate response do not occur smoothly, as they most often do in atrial fibrillation; instead, they occur in discrete "jumps," changing suddenly, for instance from 2:1 AV conduction to 3:1 or 4:1 conduction. This sort of quantum response tends to be difficult to achieve. Most often, whatever the atrial tachyarrhythmia, a combination of drugs is required (calcium blockers plus beta blockers and/or digoxin) to achieve an adequate heart rate response.

Both oral verapamil and oral diltiazem are effective in chronic heart rate management. In the acute setting, intravenous infusions of diltiazem have proven to be very effective in controlling heart rate during atrial tachycardias.

Multifocal Atrial Tachycardia: Multifocal atrial tachycardia is almost exclusively seen during acute illness, most often during acute respiratory decompensation. The arrhythmia is currently thought to be mediated by afterdepolarizations. Accordingly, verapamil can sometimes improve the arrhythmia itself instead of merely increasing the degree of AV block.

AV Nodal Reentry and Macroreentrant Tachycardias: Reentrant arrhythmias that use the AV node as part of the reentrant circuit are very susceptible to therapy with calcium blockers. Calcium blockers terminate such arrhythmias by slowing AV nodal depolarization and increasing refractoriness. As a result, *Mobitz I AV block* occurs (second-degree AV block characterized by a progressive prolongation of AV nodal conduction before a nonconducted impulse). Since these forms of reentry require conduction through the AV node with each cycle, producing a single blocked impulse in the AV node is sufficient to terminate the arrhythmias. Verapamil by intravenous bolus is extremely effective (>90%) in terminating the arrhythmias acutely. Both verapamil and diltiazem are moderately effective in preventing recurrences of the reentrant arrhythmias.

Ventricular Tachyarrhythmias

As noted, the slow calcium channel has very little to do with depolarization of the typical myocardial cell. Accordingly, neither verapamil nor diltiazem are efficacious in treating typical reentrant ventricular tachyarrhythmias.

Two clinical syndromes have been described, however, in which verapamil has been effective in treating ventricular tachycardia. Both syndromes are characterized by a lack of organic cardiac disease. Since these patients do not have the substrate for reentrant ventricular arrhythmias (i.e., myocardial disease) and since they commonly respond to verapamil (and often to beta blockers), it has been hypothesized that the arrhythmias are caused by triggered activity.

Exercise-Triggered Ventricular Tachycardia: During exercise, the patients develop sustained ventricular tachycardia that typically has left bundle branch block, right axis morphology. The arrhythmias usually respond to beta blockers. Verapamil has been reported to be effective in many of these patients.

Idiopathic Ventricular Tachycardia: Idiopathic ventricular tachycardia with right bundle branch block and left axis deviation is another arrhythmia that occurs in young patients without organic heart disease. It responds to verapamil in many patients, but its response to beta blockers has been poor.

Both syndromes are rare. The key to their diagnosis is the absence of underlying heart disease. Ventricular arrhythmias in the setting of no underlying myocardial disease are likely to be a result of some mechanism other than typical reentry.

TOXICITY AND DRUG INTERACTIONS

Verapamil has significant negative inotropic properties and can precipitate congestive heart failure in patients with impaired ventricular function. Like any calcium blocker (many of which are marketed solely for the treatment of hypertension), verapamil can produce significant hypotension. Other side effects include constipation, dizziness, nausea, headache, edema, and bradyarrhythmias (seen almost exclusively in patients with underlying SA nodal or AV conduction disease). Hypotension can be additive when verapamil is used with other antihypertensive agents. Negative inotropic effects can be additive when verapamil is given with flecainide, disopyramide, or beta blockers. Verapamil can increase drug levels of carbamazipine, cyclosporin, and theophylline. Rifampin and phenobarbital can reduce levels of verapamil. Verapamil can reduce serum lithium levels in patients taking lithium; on the other hand, verapamil can increase sensitivity to lithium.

Diltiazem also has negative inotropic properties but clinically significant impairment of ventricular function caused by diltiazem has been rare. Similar to verapamil, diltiazem can produce bradyarrhythmias and hypotension. Elevations in hepatic transaminases have been reported. Other side effects are dermatitis, headache, dizziness, and weakness.

The side effects of bradycardia, hypotension and, possibly, deterioration of ventricular function can be additive when diltiazem is used with beta blockers or antihypertensive agents. Cimetidine and ranitidine can increase diltiazem levels. Diltiazem can increase levels of digoxin, cyclosporine, and carbamazepine.

Unclassified
Antiarrhythmic Agents

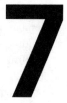

Digoxin, adenosine, and magnesium are often used to treat cardiac arrhythmias. Since these agents do not fit the Vaughan-Williams classification system (see Chapter 2), they are considered separately in this chapter.

DIGOXIN

Digitalis preparations have been used in clinical medicine since the 1700s. Digoxin, the preparation of digitalis now most commonly used, is well absorbed, is excreted by the kidneys, and has an elimination half-life of 1.7 days.

The clinical utility of digoxin is twofold. First, it increases intracellular calcium during muscle contraction, thus increasing inotropy. Second, it increases parasympathetic tone, which makes it useful for treating supraventricular arrhythmias.

Since parasympathetic innervation is greatest in the sinoatrial (SA) and atrioventricular (AV) nodes, they are the structures most affected by digoxin. Thus, digoxin can be beneficial in any arrhythmia in which the AV node plays a critical role, such as AV nodal reentrant tachycardia (in which the AV node is a direct participant in the arrhythmia itself) and in atrial fibrillation and atrial flutter. In atrial fibrillation and flutter, digitalis has little or no direct effect on the arrhythmia itself but can be useful in slowing the ventricular response by increasing the refractory period of the AV node. Digoxin can also be of benefit in treating bypass-tract-mediated tachycardias, but because the drug can have a direct effect on the bypass tract itself (resulting in a shortening of refractoriness and thus potentially making the bypass tract more dangerous), it is rarely used for these arrhythmias.

Digoxin is a very well-tolerated drug, as long as toxic levels are avoided. Digitalis toxicity, however, can be a serious clinical problem manifested by gastrointestinal symptoms (nausea, vomiting, anorexia, diarrhea, cramps), neurologic symptoms (visual disturbances, restlessness, delirium), and significant arrhythmias (SA nodal dysfunction, AV block, atrial tachycardia, junctional tachycardia, ventricular tachycardia). The cardiac arrhythmias associated with digoxin toxicity are potentially life-threatening. Digoxin toxicity appears to increase the risk of developing refractory ventricular arrhythmias or bradyarrhythmias after direct current (DC) cardioversion; cardioversion should be avoided if digoxin levels are high. The manifestations of digoxin toxicity are exacerbated by hypokalemia, and maintaining normal serum potassium levels in patients taking this drug is important.

Management of digoxin toxicity consists of stopping the drug, correcting electrolyte disturbances (especially hypokalemia and hypomagnesemia), pacing (if significant bradyarrhythmias are present), and using phenytoin or lidocaine for ventricular arrhythmias. If life-threatening arrhythmias are present, use of digoxin-specific antibodies can be rapidly effective and should be considered.

Digoxin levels can be elevated by concomitant use of quinidine, amiodarone, verapamil, erythromycin, and tetracycline. Digoxin levels can be lowered by cholestyramine and neomycin.

ADENOSINE

Adenosine is a naturally occurring nucleoside that, in high concentration, has a profound but fleeting depressive effect on the SA and AV nodes. When given intravenously, the effect of adenosine is maximal after 10 to 30 seconds and is manifested by transient high-degree AV block, profound slowing of the SA node, or both. Transient AV block is the mechanism by which the drug terminates supraventricular tachyarrhythmias (Figure 7.1). The drug is removed from the circulation very quickly; its half-life is less than 10 seconds. In addition to its electrophysiologic effects, adenosine can have a potent vasodilatory effect, but this effect is also fleeting.

Adenosine has proven very useful for the acute termination of reentrant tachyarrhythmias that involve the AV node. Almost 100% of AV nodal reentrant tachycardias and bypass-tract-mediated macroreentry can be terminated by an intravenous bolus of adeno-

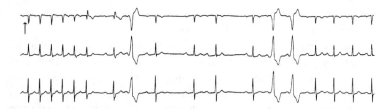

Figure 7.1. Termination of supraventricular tachycardia with adenosine. The figure illustrates termination of an episode of AV nodal reentrant tachycardia by administration of a bolus of intravenous adenosine. Surface ECG leads V1, II, and V5 are shown, top to bottom, respectively. Within seconds of administering adenosine (arrow), tachycardia abruptly terminates.

Table 7.1. Effect of Adenosine on Various Tachyarrhythmias

Termination	Transient Slowing of Heart Rate	No Response
SA nodal reentry	Atrial tachycardia	Ventricular tachycardia
AV nodal reentry	Atrial fibrillation	
Macroreentrant SVT	Atrial flutter	

SVT = supraventricular tachycardia.

sine. The drug is also helpful in diagnosing the mechanism of wide-QRS complex tachycardia—it terminates AV nodal and macroreentrant arrhythmias; causes transient heart block, which transiently slows atrial tachyarrhythmias; and generally has no effect on ventricular tachycardia (Table 7.1).

The drug is given as a rapid intravenous bolus, usually beginning with 6 mg intravenously for 1 to 2 seconds. A 12-mg bolus can be used if no effect occurs within 2 minutes.

Adenosine often causes transient bradyarrhythmias. Flushing, headache, sweating, and dizziness are also relatively common, but these symptoms last for less than 1 minute. Rare cases of exacerbation of asthma have been reported with adenosine.

MAGNESIUM

Magnesium has not received as much attention as other electrolytes, which reflects a general, recurrent theme and shortcoming in science—if something is difficult to measure, it tends to be ignored despite its potential importance. Not only is the metabolism of magnesium complicated (absorption from the gut is highly variable and depends on the level of magnesium in the diet, and the renal excretion of magnesium is also difficult to study) but serum levels of magnesium only poorly reflect body stores. Thus, there is no simple test to assess the status of a patient's magnesium stores.

Recently, however, there has been growing interest in the use of intravenous magnesium to treat a variety of medical conditions (in addition to its traditional place in the treatment of preeclampsia): asthma, ischemic heart disease, and cardiac arrhythmias. The most well-established use for parenteral magnesium is treatment of arrhythmias.

The precise mechanism by which magnesium can ameliorate arrhythmias has not been established. That magnesium might have an effect on cardiac electrophysiology is not surprising, however, when one considers that among the many enzyme systems in which magnesium plays a crucial role is the sodium–potassium pump. Magnesium can thus have an important influence on sodium and potassium transport across the cell membrane and therefore on cardiac action potential.

The most well-established use of magnesium as an antiarrhythmic agent is therapy of torsades de pointes. Most likely, magnesium has a suppressive effect on the development of afterdepolarizations responsible for this arrhythmia. Whatever the mechanism, because of its efficacy, rapidity of action, and relative safety, intravenous magnesium has become the drug of first choice in the acute treatment of torsades. Magnesium appears to be effective in this condition even when there is no evidence of magnesium depletion.

Magnesium may also have a role to play in treating arrhythmias associated with digitalis toxicity. The inhibition of the sodium–potassium pump mediated by digoxin (which may play a role in digitalis-toxic arrhythmias) appears to be countered by magnesium administration. Indeed, magnesium deficiency itself may play a role in the genesis of the arrhythmias because digoxin tends to cause magnesium wasting.

Because magnesium slows conduction in the AV node, some have reported terminating supraventricular tachyarrhythmias by giving intravenous magnesium. Although one would expect magnesium to be most effective in terminating arrhythmias in which the AV node plays a crucial role, there are a few reports suggesting that magnesium can sometimes also terminate multifocal atrial

Table 7.2. Symptoms of Magnesium Toxicity

Serum Mg++ Levels (mEq/liter)	Symptoms
5–10	ECG changes (increased PR interval and QRS duration)
10–15	Loss of reflexes
15–20	Respiratory paralysis
20–25	Cardiac arrest

ECG = electrocardiogram.

tachycardia. Magnesium administration may also help prevent postoperative arrhythmias after cardiac surgery.

Whether magnesium deficiency is a prerequisite for benefit from the intravenous administration of magnesium is not clear. Still, magnesium deficiency can cause or exacerbate cardiac arrhythmias (and cause tremors, tetany, seizures, potassium depletion, and psychiatric disturbances), so it is important to take a patient's magnesium stores into account when treating arrhythmias. A low serum magnesium level often reflects low magnesium stores, but low total magnesium may exist in the absence of hypomagnesemia. Thus, one needs to have a high index of suspicion for magnesium depletion. Especially if symptoms compatible with magnesium depletion are present, magnesium therapy should be considered in patients presenting with malnutrition, alcohol abuse, diabetes, hypokalemia, hypocalcemia, and in patients taking amphotericin B, cyclosporine, digoxin, gentamicin, loop diuretics, or pentamidine.

For the acute treatment of cardiac arrhythmias, the administration of intravenous magnesium has proven very safe. There is some potential of pushing magnesium levels into the toxic range in the presence of severe renal failure, but the overall risk of doing so is low (symptoms associated with toxic magnesium levels are listed in Table 7.2). Eight to 16 mEq of magnesium (1–2 g magnesium sulfate) can be infused rapidly during several minutes. A total of 32 mEq (4 g) can be given during 1 hour if necessary. Oral therapy is inappropriate for the acute treatment of cardiac arrhythmias because of the variable (and limited) absorption of magnesium from the gastrointestinal tract. Chronic oral administration of magnesium salts may be helpful in some conditions, such as in patients receiving loop diuretics.

Common Adverse Events with Antiarrhythmic Drugs

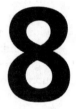

The decision to use an antiarrhythmic drug always exposes the patient to at least some risk of an adverse outcome. This chapter considers in detail three varieties of adverse events that are common to many antiarrhythmic drugs: proarrhythmia, drug-drug interactions, and drug-device interactions.

PROARRHYTHMIA

It may seem paradoxical that drugs designed to suppress cardiac arrhythmias may instead worsen them or cause arrhythmias that did not previously exist. Proarrhythmia begins to make sense, however, when one considers that most arrhythmias ultimately are caused by some change in cardiac action potential, and that most antiarrhythmic drugs work by causing changes in the cardiac action potential. One always hopes that the changes caused by drugs make arrhythmias less likely to occur. However, one must accept that the opposite might happen.

At least four categories of drug-induced proarrhythmic can be seen: bradyarrhythmias, worsening of reentry, torsades de pointes, and arrhythmias resulting from worsening hemodynamics.

Bradyarrhythmias

Antiarrhythmic drugs can abnormally slow the heart rate by suppressing the sinoatrial (SA) node or by causing atrioventricular (AV) block. Generally speaking, however, only patients who already have underlying disease in the SA node, AV node, or His-Purkinje system are likely to experience symptomatic slowing of the heart rate with antiarrhythmic drugs.

Sinus bradycardia can be seen with any drug that suppresses the SA node—beta blockers, calcium blockers, or digitalis. Again, however, symptomatic sinus slowing is almost never seen in patients who do not have underlying SA nodal dysfunction. The most common example of drug-induced symptomatic sinus slowing (and probably the most common cause of syncope in patients with SA nodal dysfunction) is the prolonged pause that can be seen when a drug is used to convert atrial fibrillation. The phenomenon occurs because diseased SA nodes display the property of overdrive suppression of automaticity—any atrial tachycardia suppresses SA nodal automaticity. As a result, when the atrial tachycardia suddenly stops, it can take many seconds for the diseased SA node to begin firing again, and during that time the patient is asystolic. Unfortunately, SA nodal disease is relatively common in patients with atrial tachyarrhythmias because the two are often part of the same disease process—both are caused by diffuse fibrotic changes in the atria. This form of bradycardia is related to antiarrhythmic drugs in that it is the drug resultant that stops the tachycardia—the pause itself is not a drug effect.

AV nodal block can occur when beta blockers, calcium blockers, digoxin, or any combination of these drugs are used in patients with underlying AV nodal disease. Digitalis toxicity is the most common cause of drug-induced AV nodal block.

Class IA, Class IC, or occasionally Class III drugs can produce block in the His-Purkinje system in patients who have underlying distal conducting system disease. Because subsidiary pacemakers distal to the His bundle are unreliable when distal heart block occurs, antiarrhythmic drugs should be used with particular care in patients with known or suspected distal conducting-system disease.

In general, the treatment of drug-induced bradyarrhythmias is to discontinue the offending agent and use temporary or permanent pacemakers as necessary to maintain adequate heart rate.

Worsening of Reentrant Arrhythmias

Figure 8.1 reviews how antiarrhythmic drugs can work to benefit reentrant arrhythmias. By changing the conduction velocity, refractoriness, or both in various parts of the reentrant circuit, antiarrhythmic drugs can eliminate the critical relationships necessary to initiate and sustain reentry.

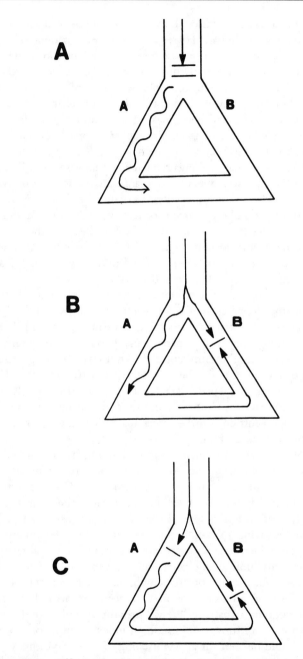

Figure 8.1. Effect of antiarrhythmic drugs on a reentrant circuit (same figure as Figure 2.3).

Chapter 2 discussed how antiarrhythmic drugs can worsen reentrant arrhythmias. To review, consider a patient who has an occult reentrant circuit whose electrophysiologic properties do not support a reentrant arrhythmia. Giving the patient mexiletine, a drug that reduces refractory periods, may reduce the refractory period of one pathway, giving this circuit the characteristics shown in Figure 8.1A, and thus making a reentrant arrhythmia much more likely to occur. A similar scenario can be developed for a patient with the circuit shown in Figure 8.1C and who is given sotalol, a drug that prolongs refractory periods (see also Figure 2.3).

Unfortunately, whenever an antiarrhythmic drug is given to a patient with a potential reentrant circuit, the drug may render an arrhythmia less likely to occur or it may render an arrhythmia *more* likely to occur. This sad truth follows because the very same mechanism that produces an antiarrhythmic effect (namely, the alteration of conduction velocity and refractory periods) is also the mechanism that produces a proarrhythmic effect.

Exacerbation of reentrant tachycardias can occur whether one is treating supraventricular or ventricular arrhythmias. The frequency is highest with Class IC drugs (since profound slowing of conduction velocity is a particularly good way to potentiate reentry), but it is also fairly common with Class IA drugs. Exacerbation of reentry can also be seen with Class IB and Class III drugs, but with less frequency. Class II and Class IV drugs rarely produce worsening of reentrant arrhythmias and usually only in patients with supraventricular arrhythmias that utilize the AV node as part of the reentrant circuit.

Clinically, this form of proarrhythmia is manifested by an increase in the frequency or duration of a reentrant arrhythmia. Not uncommonly, and especially with Class IC drugs, a reentrant arrhythmia becomes relatively incessant. Since the drugs most commonly producing this sort of proarrhythmia (Class IA and Class IC) cause a slowing in conduction velocity, often the proarrhythmic tachycardia occurs at a slower rate than did the original tachycardia. If the arrhythmia being exacerbated is ventricular tachycardia, the clinical manifestation of proarrhythmia may be sudden death.

Treating an exacerbation of a reentrant arrhythmia requires the recognition that the "new" arrhythmia is drug-induced. This recognition, in turn, requires a high index of suspicion. In general, one should be alert for any worsening of the arrhythmia whenever one is treating a reentrant arrhythmia with antiarrhythmic drugs. If proarrhythmia is suspected, the offending drugs should be immediately stopped, and the patient supported hemodynamically until the drug metabolizes (a particular problem when using a drug with a long half-life). Proarrhythmic reentry, like spontaneous reentry, can often be terminated by antitachycardia pacing techniques. If needed, a temporary pacemaker can be placed for antitachycardia pacing until the patient stabilizes. Adding additional antiarrhythmic drugs when this type of proarrhythmia is present often makes things worse and should be avoided if possible.

Torsades de Pointes

Torsades de pointes is the name given to the polymorphic ventricular tachycardias associated with prolonged QT intervals or other repolarization abnormalities. As outlined in Chapter 1, these arrhythmias are thought to be caused by the development of afterdepolarizations, which, in turn, are a common result of using antiarrhythmic drugs.

Drugs that increase the duration of the cardiac action potential—Class IA and Class III drugs—can produce the pause-dependent ventricular tachyarrhythmias that are mediated by early afterdepolarizations (EADs). As shown in Chapter 1 (see Figure 1.16), the arrhythmias generally present as frequent, recurrent bursts of polymorphous ventricular tachycardia preceded by a pause. They are often relatively asymptomatic, but they can also produce syncope or death.

Proarrhythmia caused by this mechanism should be strongly suspected whenever a patient treated with quinidine, procainamide, disopyramide, or sotalol complains of episodes of lightheadedness or syncope. In the case of sotalol, the risk of torsades is directly related to the degree of QT interval prolongation—the longer the QT interval, the higher the risk. Such an association is much less clear with Class IA drugs. The incidence of torsades with Class IA or Class III drugs is generally estimated to be at least 2%–5%.

Toxic levels of digoxin can produce polymorphic ventricular tachycardia by causing DADs (see Figure 1.15B). This type of arrhythmia is not pause dependent. A new onset of polymorphic ventricular tachycardia or the development of syncope in patients treated with digoxin should prompt measurement of a digoxin level.

Worsening of Hemodynamics

Much less well documented are the arrhythmias that occur as a result of drug-induced cardiac decompensation or hypotension.

Acute cardiac failure can lead directly to arrhythmias by causing abnormal automaticity (ICU arrhythmias). Hypotension can cause arrhythmias by the same mechanism or by causing reflex sympathetic stimulation. Thus, antiarrhythmic drugs that decrease the inotropic state of the heart (beta blockers, calcium blockers, disopyramide, or flecainide) or drugs that cause vasodilation (calcium blockers, some beta blockers, and the intravenous administration of quinidine, procainamide, bretylium, or amiodarone) can occasionally lead to cardiac arrhythmias.

Proarrhythmia in Perspective

Although the potential for antiarrhythmic drugs to worsen cardiac arrhythmias has been known for decades, the potential magnitude of the problem has been recognized for only a few years. The single most important event that drew attention to the problem of proarrhythmia was the reporting of the results of the Cardiac Arrhythmia Suppression Trial (CAST). In CAST, survivors of myocardial infarction who had reduced left ventricular ejection fractions and complex ventricular ectopy were randomized to placebo or to one of three antiarrhythmic drugs (encainide, flecainide, or moricizine) that had been shown previously to suppress their ectopy. The hypothesis of the study was that suppressing ambient ectopy would improve the mortality of the patients. Instead, the results showed that patients treated with encainide or flecainide had a fourfold *increase* in the risk of sudden death (patients treated with moricizine showed no benefit from drug treatment) and had a significant increase in overall mortality. The increase in risk for fatal arrhythmias was not limited to the first few days or weeks of drug therapy but persisted throughout the follow-up period.

CAST proved to be a major blow to the Class IC drugs in particular, but evidence suggests that its results might also apply, at least to some extent, to other antiarrhythmic agents. Other trials have suggested, for instance, that both use of quinidine for atrial fibrillation and use of Class I drugs in survivors of myocardial infarction have produced significant increases in mortality.

As a result, most electrophysiologists have become convinced that the proarrhythmic effects of Class I drugs outweigh the antiarrhythmic effects, at least in patients with underlying heart disease. Lately, it has been fashionable in some circles to extol the relative virtues of Class III drugs, but these drugs, too, carry a significant risk of proarrhythmia (sotalol and ibutilide are especially efficient at causing torsades).

Using antiarrhythmic drugs always involves the risk of making heart rhythm worse instead of better. (For each drug, the relative risks of causing the major forms of proarrhythmia are shown in Table 8.1). One should prescribe these drugs only if it is necessary for prolongation of survival or for amelioration of significant symptomatology. Most important, whenever one is compelled to prescribe antiarrhythmic drugs, one should feel obligated to do whatever possible to minimize the risk of symptomatic or life-threatening proarrhythmia.

Since reentrant ventricular tachycardia (and therefore drug-induced worsening of reentry) generally is seen only in the presence of underlying cardiac disease, one must be especially cautious about using antiarrhythmic drugs in patients with heart disease. When prescribing antiarrhythmic drugs in this setting, one must make sure that serum electrolytes (especially potassium) are kept well within the normal range. In addition, cardiac function should be optimized because hemodynamic compromise can worsen arrhythmias. Cardiac ischemia should be managed aggressively. Not only does ischemia itself precipitate arrhythmias, but ischemia also renders drug-induced proarrhythmia more likely.

Table 8.1. Relative Risk of Drug-Induced Proarrhythmia

Drug	Risk of Exacerbation of Reentry	Risk of Torsades de Pointes
Class IA		
Quinidine	+ +	+ +
Procainamide	+ +	+ +
Disopyramide	+ +	+ +
Class IB		
Lidocaine	+	0
Mexiletine	+	0
Phenytoin	+	0
Class IC		
Flecainide	+ + +	0
Propafenone	+ + +	0
Moricizine	+ + +	+
Class III		
Amiodarone	+	+
Bretylium	+	+
Sotalol	+	+ + +
Ibutilide	+ +	+ + +

Torsades de pointes probably occurs in an otherwise normal subset of the population at large—a subset of individuals who are prone to develop afterdepolarizations whenever something acts to prolong cardiac action potentials. Thus, underlying heart disease is not necessary for this form of proarrhythmia—any patient treated with a Class IA or Class III drug is a candidate for torsades. Patients started on therapy with such drugs should be placed on a cardiac monitor for several days because torsades is most often first seen during the initial 3 or 4 days of therapy (although it can occur any time). With sotalol, the QT interval should be monitored carefully during drug loading. Serum potassium levels should also be watched carefully; in fact, one should use torsades-producing agents with trepidation in patients requiring potassium-wasting diuretics.

DRUG-DRUG INTERACTIONS

Antiarrhythmic drugs seem to produce more than their share of interactions with other drugs. Interactions generally are related to competition with other drugs for serum proteins on which to bind or to drug-induced changes in hepatic metabolism. The major interactions between antiarrhythmic drugs and other agents (see the discussions of the individual antiarrhythmic drugs) are summarized in Table 8.2.

DRUG-DEVICE INTERACTIONS

Antiarrhythmic drugs can occasionally interfere with the function of electronic pacemakers and implantable cardioverter defibrillators (ICDs). It is relatively rare for antiarrhythmic drugs to significantly interfere with pacemakers. Class IA drugs can increase pacing thresholds, but only at toxic drug levels. Class IC drugs, sotalol, and amiodarone can increase pacing thresholds at therapeutic levels, but only rarely to a clinically important extent. The effects of antiarrhythmic drugs on pacing thresholds are summarized in Table 8.3. The interaction of antiarrhythmic drugs with ICDs can occur in several ways and is often clinically significant. Two major problems caused by antiarrhythmic drugs are that they can change the energy required for successful defibrillation, and they can change the characteristics of the arrhythmia being treated.

The effect of antiarrhythmic drugs on defibrillation energy requirements is an important consideration because increasing the defibrillation threshold can render an ICD ineffective. The effects

Table 8.2. Major Drug Interactions of Antiarrhythmic Drugs

Drug	Levels Increased	Levels Decreased	Levels or Effect Increased	Levels or Effect Decreased
Class IA				
Quinidine	Amiodarone	Phenobarbital Phenytoin Rifampin	Anticholinergics Warfarin Phenothiazines Digoxin	
Procainamide	Amiodarone Trimethoprim Cimetidine	Ethanol		
Disopyramide		Phenobarbital Phenytoin Rifampin		
Class IB				
Lidocaine	Propranolol Metoprolol Cimetidine	Phenobarbital		
Mexiletine	Cimetidine Choramphenicol Isoniazid	Phenytoin Phenobarbital Rifampin	Theophylline Lidocaine Phenytoin	
Phenytoin	Cimetidine Isoniazid Sulfonamides Amiodarone	Theophylline	Theophylline Quinidine Disopyramide Lidocaine Mexiletine	
Class IC				
Flecainide	Amiodarone Cimetidine Propranolol Quinidine		Digoxin	
Propafenone	Cimetidine Quinidine	Phenobarbital Phenytoin Rifampin	Digoxin Propranolol Metoprolol Theophylline Cyclosporine Desipramine Warfarin	
Moricizine	Cimetidine			Theophylline
Class III				
Amiodarone			Warfarin Digoxin Class I drugs Beta blockers Calcium blockers	
Sotalol			Class IA drugs* Beta blockers	
Ibutilide			Class IA drugs*	

* Produce additive risk of torsades.

Table 8.3. Effect of Antiarrhythmic Drugs on Pacing Thresholds

Increase at Normal Drug Levels	Increase at Toxic Drug Levels	No increase
Flecainide	Quinidine	Lidocaine
Propafenone	Procainamide	Mexiletine
Amiodarone	Disopyramide	
Sotalol		

Table 8.4. Effect of Antiarrhythmic Drugs on Defibrillation Thresholds

Increase	Mixed effect	Decrease
Flecainide	Quinidine	Sotalol
Propafenone	Procainamide	Bretylium
Lidocaine	Amiodarone	
Mexiletine		

of various drugs on defibrillations energy requirements are summarized in Table 8.4. In general, drugs that block the sodium channel increase defibrillation energy requirements (thus, Class IC drugs have the most profound effect, and Class IA and Class IB drugs tend to have proportionally lesser effects), and drugs that block the potassium channels (e.g., sotalol) decrease defibrillation energy requirements. Drugs that affect both the sodium and potassium channels (i.e., Class IA drugs and amiodarone) have mixed effects—sometimes they increase and sometimes they decrease defibrillation energy requirements. If one must prescribe a drug that has the potential of increasing defibrillation energy requirements for a patient who has an ICD, one should retest defibrillation thresholds after the drug has been loaded to be sure the ICD is still capable of delivering sufficient energy to reliably defibrillate the patient.

Antiarrhythmic drugs can also interact with ICDs by changing the characteristics of a patient's ventricular tachycardia. By slowing the rate of ventricular tachycardia, a drug can render the arrhythmia more amenable to antitachycardia pacing, which potentially makes the ICD more effective. On the other hand, by slowing the rate of ventricular tachycardia below the recognition rate of the ICD, a drug can cause the ICD to fail to recognize (and therefore fail to treat) recurrent arrhythmias. Antiarrhythmic drugs can also cause reentrant ventricular arrhythmias to recur more frequently or even to become incessant, thus inducing frequent ICD therapy, which, in turn, can cause excessive discomfort and premature battery depletion of the ICD. In general, when one is compelled to add an antiarrhythmic drug to the treatment regimen of a patient with an ICD, one should consider electrophysiologic testing to reexamine the characteristics of the patient's arrhythmias and to be sure the ICD is optimally programmed to treat the arrhythmias.

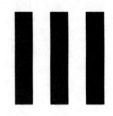

Antiarrhythmic Drugs in the Treatment of Cardiac Arrhythmias

Basic Principles of Using Antiarrhythmic Drugs

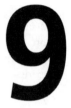

The first two sections of the book concerned the mechanisms of cardiac arrhythmias, the mechanism of action of antiarrhythmic drugs, and the features of specific antiarrhythmic drugs. In the final section, that information is applied to the use of antiarrhythmic drugs in the treatment of specific cardiac arrhythmias. Chapter 9 reviews some basic principles of using antiarrhythmic drugs.

On the basis of the generally limited efficacy of antiarrhythmic drugs and of their inherent propensity to cause serious problems, the first principle should be completely self-evident; namely, one should avoid using antiarrhythmic drugs whenever possible. Thus, when one has decided to prescribe an antiarrhythmic drug, the final step before actually writing the order should be to ask, "Does this patient really need this drug?" There are only two general conditions in which using an antiarrhythmic drug is entirely appropriate: when an arrhythmia is potentially life-threatening and when an arrhythmia is significantly symptomatic. Before prescribing an antiarrhythmic drug, the physician should be certain that the arrhythmia meets one of the two conditions.

The second basic principle is to keep the goal of treatment clearly in mind and to tailor the aggressiveness of one's therapy accordingly. If one is treating an arrhythmia to prevent death, for instance, an aggressive approach is often appropriate and necessary—one must not relax until the risk of death has been optimally suppressed. On the other hand, if one is treating an arrhythmia to relieve symptoms, a more circumspect approach is appropriate. In this instance, one generally should use a stepwise strategy, beginning with milder, less risky forms of treatment, and reassessing the risk-benefit ratio before each potential escalation of therapy. Most grievous errors made in using antiarrhythmic drugs are related to a muddling of the two distinct treatment goals. All too often physicians tread lightly when faced with a life-threatening arrhythmia; or worse, they pursue insignificant arrhythmias with Ninja-like intensity. Either error can result in unnecessary injury or death.

The final basic principle of using antiarrhythmic drugs is that, if one feels compelled to expose a patient to the risk of the drugs, one should also feel compelled to take every reasonable precaution to reduce the risks. Given the almost universal risk of proarrhythmia, one should strongly consider placing patients on a cardiac monitor while antiarrhythmic drugs are being initiated because, although proarrhythmia can occur any time during the course of treatment, a significant proportion of these events occur during the first 3 or 4 days of drug usage. Most important, one must take great care in deciding which drug to use. The choice must be individualized. The accompanying tables summarize the factors that should be considered in choosing antiarrhythmic drugs for patients with and without significant underlying cardiac disease.

One should avoid using drugs that are plainly contraindicated for particular patients. Procainamide, for instance, should not be used in patients with systemic lupus erythematosus; quinidine should not be used in patients with chronic colitis; patients with severe lung disease (in whom mild pulmonary toxicity goes a long way) ideally should not receive amiodarone; patients with a history of heart failure should not receive drugs with negative inotropic effects. Beyond these obvious individual considerations, the presence or absence of underlying heart disease is the most important variable in choosing an antiarrhythmic drug because heart disease predisposes one to reentrant circuits and, therefore, to proarrhythmia. As shown in Table 9.1, beta blockers and Class IB drugs are the safest choice regardless of whether the patient has underlying heart disease. Class IC drugs are reasonably safe for patients with normal hearts, but because of the frequency with which Class IC drugs exacerbate reentrant arrhythmias, they are completely unacceptable in patients with underlying cardiac disease. Class IA drugs carry a moderate risk of toxicity for patients without cardiac disease because they cause both torsades and end-organ toxicity; for patients with cardiac disease, a moderate risk of exacerbation of reentrant arrhythmias must be added. Sotalol carries a moderate risk of torsades for all patients and a risk of exacerbating heart failure for patients with underlying disease. Amiodarone carries a substantial risk of end-organ toxicity for all patients.

Table 9.1. Relative Overall Risk of Serious Toxicity from Antiarrhythmic Drugs[a]

Increasing Order of Risk for Patients with no Underlying Heart Disease	Increasing Order of Risk for Patients with Underlying Heart Disease
Class II	Class II
Class IB	Class IB
Class IC	Sotalol
Sotalol	Amiodarone
Class IA	Class IA
Amiodarone[b]	Class IC (should not use)[c]

[a] Ranking of relative risks takes into account both the risk of proarrhythmia and the risk of end-organ toxicity.

[b] For patients without underlying heart disease, the impressive range of end-organ toxicity makes amiodarone the riskiest drug.

[c] For patients with end-organ toxicity, the ranking changes because these patients have a much higher propensity for proarrhythmia. Class IC drugs should virtually never be used in these patients.

Table 9.2 ranks the efficacy of antiarrhythmic drugs for atrial and ventricular tachyarrhythmias and for AV node-dependent arrhythmias. For atrial tachyarrhythmias, Class IA drugs and sotalol are roughly equal in efficacy. Class IC drugs and amiodarone are somewhat more effective than are Class IA drugs, and Class IB drugs have virtually no efficacy for these arrhythmias. Most antiarrhythmic agents have some degree of efficacy against AV node-dependent arrhythmias. For ventricular tachyarrhythmias, Class II and Class IB drugs are least effective; amiodarone is most effective.

Table 9.3 synthesizes the data from Tables 9.1 and 9.2 to generalize about the potential drugs of choice for atrial and ventricular tachyarrhythmias (albeit drug selection must be individualized in every case). The main consideration is always to balance efficacy with safety.

The drug of choice in treating both atrial and ventricular tachyarrhythmias depends on the presence or absence of underlying cardiac disease. For instance, in the absence of heart disease, Class IC drugs may offer the most favorable balance of efficacy and safety in the treatment of atrial tachyarrhythmias; in the presence of underlying heart disease, Class IC agents (because of their impressive propensity to exacerbate reentrant ventricular arrhythmias)

Table 9.2. Relative Efficacy of Antiarrhythmic Drugs for Tachyarrhythmias[a]

Atrial Tachyarrhythmias[b]	AVN-Dependent Tachyarrhythmias[c]	Ventricular Tachyarrhythmias
Class IA	Class IA	Class II
Sotalol	Digoxin	Class IB
Class IC	Class II	Class IA
Amiodarone	Verapamil[d]	Class IC
	Sotalol	Sotalol
	Class IC	Amiodarone
	Amiodarone	
	Verapamil[e]	
	Adenosine[e]	

[a] Drugs are listed in order of increasing efficacy.
[b] Atrial tachycardia, atrial fibrillation, atrial flutter.
[c] AV-nodal reentry, macroreentry (bypass-tract-mediated).
[d] When used orally for maintenance of sinus rhythm.
[e] When used intravenously for acute termination of the arrhythmia.

Table 9.3. Drugs of Choice for Atrial and Ventricular Arrhythmias[a]

Underlying Heart Disease Absent		Underlying Heart Disease Present	
Atrial Arrhythmias[b]	Ventricular Arrhythmias[c]	Atrial Arrhythmias	Ventricular Arrhythmias
Class IC	Class II	Sotalol	Amiodarone
Sotalol	Class IB	Amiodarone	Sotalol
Class IA	Sotalol	Class IA	Class IA
	Class IC		
	Class IA		
	Amiodarone		

[a] Drugs are listed in decreasing order of choice.
[b] Atrial tachycardia, atrial fibrillation, atrial flutter.
[c] Complex ventricular ectopy, ventricular tachycardia, ventricular fibrillation.

should never be used. For ventricular arrhythmias, the primary consideration in patients without underlying heart disease (i.e., patients in whom the risk for sudden death is usually very low) is not to increase the risk of death by exposing the patients to the risk of proarrhythmia. Thus, in choosing drug therapy one should err on the side of safety—Class II and Class IB drugs should be considered despite their limited effectiveness. As soon as one moves beyond these two classes of drugs, one begins accepting a substantial risk of proarrhythmia or other significant toxicity. On the other hand, for patients with underlying heart disease who require therapy for ventricular arrhythmias, efficacy is the primary consideration. In these patients, insufficient efficacy is likely to be manifested by sudden death. Thus, amiodarone is often the first drug considered despite its potential for causing long-term toxicity. In Table 9.3, for drugs listed as secondary choices after amiodarone, not only do the odds of efficacy decrease but the risk of proarrhythmia increases.

In summary, when it comes to using antiarrhythmic drugs there are no pretty choices. The best choice is to avoid them altogether. If this is not possible, one must proceed with the goals of treatment clearly in mind and take every precaution to avoid producing more problems than the ones being treated.

Treatment of Supraventricular Tachyarrhythmias

10

Traditionally, clinicians have tended to divide the supraventricular tachyarrhythmias into two broad categories: paroxysmal atrial tachycardia (PAT) and atrial flutter/fibrillation. The term PAT has fallen into disfavor of late (it is an artifact of the days before the mechanisms of supraventricular arrhythmias were understood), but this bimodal categorization of supraventricular arrhythmias still lends itself nicely to a discussion of therapy.

PAROXYSMAL ATRIAL TACHYCARDIA

PAT is a term used to describe regular supraventricular tachyarrhythmias that occur with sudden onset and terminate equally suddenly. Thus, PAT is a catchall phrase that incorporates all reentrant supraventricular arrhythmias except atrial fibrillation and atrial flutter. More than 50% of PATs are caused by atrioventricular (AV) nodal reentrant tachycardia, and approximately 40% are caused by macroreentrant tachycardia mediated by an overt or concealed bypass tract. The remaining 5% to 10% are caused by reentrant atrial tachycardia or sinoatrial (SA) nodal reentrant tachycardia.

The acute and chronic therapies of PAT are listed in Table 10.1. Acute therapy is aimed at terminating an episode of PAT. In general, this is easy to achieve. Since the AV node or the SA node is an integral part of the reentrant circuit in 90% to 95% of PATs (the exception is reentrant atrial tachycardia, an arrhythmia that can

---

Table 10.1. Acute and Chronic Treatment of Paroxysmal Atrial Tachycardia

Acute Treatment

Goal: Termination of the arrhythmia

    Step 1: Vagal maneuvers such as Valsalva (may be tried by the patient before seeking medical attention)

    Step 2: Intravenous administration of adenosine or verapamil

    Termination by antitachycardia pacing or DC cardioversion (rarely necessary)

Chronic Treatment

Goal: Prevention of recurrences

    Infrequent or easy-to-terminate recurrences—no specific chronic therapy may be necessary

    Other types of recurrences

        Treatment of choice—EP testing with RF ablation to abolish reentry

        Drug therapy—one or more of several drugs may be tried empirically (see Table 9.2)

EP = electrophysiologic; RF = radiofrequency.

usually be recognized by the presence of an unusual P wave axis), maneuvers or drugs that produce transient SA nodal or AV nodal block are highly effective in terminating supraventricular arrhythmias. Many patients who have recurrent PAT can therefore terminate episodes themselves by performing maneuvers that cause a sudden increase in vagal tone. Such maneuvers include Valsalva, carotid massage, ocular massage, and dunking one's face in ice water. If pharmacologic intervention is necessary, the treatment of choice is intravenous adenosine, which is virtually always effective—in fact, if adenosine fails to terminate the arrhythmia, the diagnosis of PAT needs to be seriously reconsidered. Intravenous verapamil is also highly effective. Other AV nodal-blocking drugs (digoxin, beta blockers) are effective but have a much longer onset of action and, once loaded, their effect persists. Unless these drugs are being administered for chronic use, they are almost never given for acute treatment of PAT. Antitachycardia pacing techniques are also highly effective in terminating supraventricular arrhythmias, but since so many other less invasive options are available, pacing is rarely used unless an atrial pacemaker is already in place.

The chronic therapy for PAT has undergone a revolution. Before 1990, pharmacologic therapy was the only viable option for most patients. Although the choices of drug therapy for the chronic treatment of PAT are broad and include all AV nodal-blocking agents (beta blockers, calcium blockers and digoxin) and Class IA, Class IC, and Class III antiarrhythmic drugs, before 1990, patients would have had to take potentially toxic drugs every day to prevent non–life-threatening arrhythmias that might otherwise occur only infrequently. Given that choice, many patients quite reasonably opted for no therapy and accepted the fact that they would have to make periodic pilgrimages to emergency rooms to terminate acute episodes.

Fortunately, patients no longer have to make such a choice. When the mechanisms of the arrhythmias that cause PAT became understood, and with parallel advances in technology, virtually all forms of PAT became curable by the technique of radiofrequency ablation. With this technique, critical components of the reentrant pathways responsible for a patient's arrhythmia can be mapped in the electrophysiology catheterization laboratory and cauterized directly through the electrophysiology catheter. The success rate for curing AV nodal reentrant tachycardias and tachycardias mediated by bypass tracts is well in excess of 90%. SA nodal reentry and intra-atrial reentry can be cured with a somewhat lower rate of frequency, but these arrhythmias are rare. Today, patients with almost any form of PAT should be referred for radiofrequency ablation if chronic drug therapy of any type is being considered.

ATRIAL FIBRILLATION AND ATRIAL FLUTTER

Atrial fibrillation and atrial flutter are fundamentally different from most arrhythmias causing PAT because they arise in the atrial myocardium itself and therefore do not require either the AV node or the SA node for their initiation or continuation. Atrial fibrillation and atrial flutter can persist in the presence of a nonfunctioning SA node or complete AV block. Therefore, the measures commonly used to terminate PAT (i.e., producing transient AV nodal block through vagal maneuvers or by drug therapy) do not work with atrial fibrillation and flutter. Drugs that can terminate these arrhythmias and prevent recurrence must necessarily act on the atrial myocardium, in other words, Class IA, Class IC, and Class III antiarrhythmic drugs. Therefore, treatment is inherently difficult and relatively risky. Often, one is compelled to accept a lesser therapeutic goal than restoration and maintenance of sinus rhythm—one must be content to control only the ventricular

---

Table 10.2. Common Underlying Causes of Atrial Fibrillation and Flutter

---

Underlying heart disease
   Valvular and congenital heart disease
   Hypertensive heart disease
   Acute ischemia or infarction
   Cardiomyopathic diseases
   Pericarditis
Systemic disorders
   Hyperthyroidism
   Acute pulmonary disease
   Acute ethanol ingestion ("holiday heart")
   Stimulant administration or ingestion (e.g., caffeine, amphetamines,
      theophylline)

---

rate when the patient has chronic or recurrent atrial fibrillation or flutter.

Unlike arrhythmias that cause PAT, atrial fibrillation and atrial flutter often are related to an underlying disease process. Treating these arrhythmias, therefore, must always involve a systematic search for a primary cause. Table 10.2 lists the common underlying causes of atrial fibrillation and flutter.

Arrhythmias caused by systemic processes (electrolyte disturbances, hyperthyroidism, pulmonary disease, use of alcohol or stimulant drugs) often improve or disappear once the systemic process is addressed. Arrhythmias associated with underlying heart disease, on the other hand, often persist even when therapy of heart disease is optimized.

Prognosis

Whether the presence of atrial fibrillation and flutter affect longevity is somewhat controversial. Several studies suggest that, in the presence of underlying cardiac disease, chronic atrial fibrillation is associated with an increase in mortality. However, it is unclear whether atrial fibrillation itself increases mortality, or whether it is simply a marker of more significant underlying disease. Lone atrial fibrillation (atrial fibrillation in the absence of an identifiable underlying cause) has not been shown to be associated with an increase in mortality. Similarly, paroxysmal atrial fibrillation has not been clearly associated with decreased survival. It has not been established whether having lone atrial fibrillation and paroxysmal atrial fibrillation is inherently better than having chronic atrial fibrillation, or whether the more favorable prognoses of lone atrial fibrillation and paroxysmal atrial fibrillation are related to the fact that they are seen in younger patients.

Consequences

Atrial fibrillation and flutter have three major consequences that must be addressed in planning therapy: loss of the atrial kick, the rapid heart rate itself, and the risk of thromboembolism (Table 10.3).

Loss of Atrial Kick: The function of atrial contraction is to boost diastolic pressure within the ventricles just before ventricular systole begins. End-diastolic pressure (EDP) is of paramount importance in determining the force of ventricular contraction and therefore of ventricular stroke volume. EDP is so important that, in general, homeostatic mechanisms work to maintain it regardless of whether there is an atrial kick. The importance of the atrial kick in maintaining adequate EDP directly depends on the relative compliance, or "stiffness," of the ventricle. The atrial kick is vitally important in patients whose ventricles are noncompliant (i.e., stiff), a condition that occurs in the setting of ventricular hypertrophy, whether it has been caused by aortic stenosis, hypertension, or idiopathic

---

Table 10.3. Major Consequences of Atrial Fibrillation

Loss of atrial kick
  Major hemodynamic compromise in patients with poor LV compliance
    (i.e., patients with ventricular hypertrophy)
  Mild to moderate hemodynamic compromise in patients with normal LV
    compliance
  Minimal to mild hemodynamic compromise in patients with increased
    LV compliance (i.e., patients with dilated cardiomyopathies)
Tachycardia
  Significant symptoms (palpitations, cardiac ischemia if CAD is present)
  Tachycardiomyopathy (weakening of ventricular myocardium from
    chronic tachycardia)
Thrombus formation
  Stroke or other manifestations of thromboembolic disorder

CAD = coronary artery disease; LV = left ventricle.

hypertrophic cardiomyopathy. In these patients, very high EDP is necessary to maintain an adequate stroke volume, and the high EDP is provided, at the last instant of diastole, by the atrial kick. If the atrial kick is lost (e.g., because of the onset of atrial fibrillation), the only way to achieve adequate EDP is to raise the *mean* diastolic pressure—and this is exactly what happens. Because the heart's compensatory mechanisms attempt to maintain the EDP regardless of whether there is an atrial kick, the mean diastolic pressure suddenly rises, and pulmonary congestion ensues. Thus, patients with poor ventricular compliance develop severe symptoms almost immediately if atrial fibrillation occurs; atrial kick is vital in these patients.

On the other hand, patients with dilated cardiomyopathies have enlarged, "baggy" ventricles that are abnormally compliant. In these patients, the atrial kick contributes relatively little to EDP because the relatively small volume of blood provided by atrial contraction boosts pressure only slightly in a highly compliant ventricle. These patients tend to have relatively little change in baseline symptoms with the onset of atrial fibrillation, and they often are unable to perceive any difference between sinus rhythm and atrial fibrillation.

Patients with normal ventricles and with normal ventricular compliance tend to experience intermediate symptoms with the onset of atrial fibrillation. Their EDP is maintained by a rise in mean diastolic pressure, but generally the elevations are not sufficient to produce pulmonary edema. These patients can usually pinpoint the time of onset of atrial fibrillation, but in most cases the symptoms are limited to palpitations and perhaps a mild sensation of breathlessness.

Tachycardia: Unless the patient has AV conduction disease or is medicated with digitalis, beta blockers, or calcium-channel blockers, tachycardia ensues immediately with the onset of atrial fibrillation or flutter. How the tachycardia is perceived varies considerably from patient to patient. In general, with acute onset of the arrhythmia, the tachycardia is quite symptomatic. The transient decrease in stroke volume resulting from the loss of the atrial kick is partially compensated by an increase in sympathetic tone, which directly increases the heart rate and frequently also causes a sensation of anxiety. The anxiety, in turn, further increases sympathetic tone. Thus, it is not unusual for a patient with acute atrial fibrillation or flutter to present with very rapid heart rates, often in excess of 200 beats/min, and extreme palpitations. In general, however, sympathetic tone drops within a few hours, and the heart rate slows to a more reasonable level.

Even more disturbing than extreme acute tachycardia is the phenomenon of *tachycardiomyopathy*, which sometimes occurs with chronically elevated heart rates. Tachycardiomyopathy refers to the ventricular dysfunction that results from tachycardias that persist for weeks or months. Although relatively uncommon, this condition is indistinguishable from other forms of dilated cardiomyopathy. Fortunately, tachycardiomyopathy is largely reversible if the heart rate is brought under control. The existence of tachycardiomyopathy underscores the fact that the rapid heart rates accompanying atrial fibrillation and flutter have significance beyond merely producing palpitations.

Thromboembolism: Perhaps the major hemodynamic consequence of atrial fibrillation (and to a far lesser extent, atrial flutter) is the risk of thromboembolism. One-third of patients with chronic atrial fibrillation eventually experience stroke, and approximately 75% of the strokes are thought to be embolic in nature. Antiembolic therapy with warfarin, or to a lesser extent with aspirin, has been shown to significantly reduce the risk of stroke in patients with chronic atrial fibrillation.

THERAPY OF PAROXYSMAL ATRIAL FIBRILLATION AND ATRIAL FLUTTER

Figure 10.1 outlines acute therapy of paroxysmal atrial fibrillation and atrial flutter. Since by definition patients with paroxysmal arrhythmias usually have normal in sinus rhythm, the primary goal of therapy is to restore normal sinus rhythm and to do so within 24 hours of the onset of the arrhythmia (to avoid the likelihood of formation of atrial thrombi). In most patients, paroxysmal atrial fibrillation and flutter spontaneously convert to sinus rhythm within a few hours of onset. Thus, in most instances, one merely needs to control the heart rate and wait. If the arrhythmia persists for 24 hours, elective direct current (DC) cardioversion (or pharmacologic cardioversion) should be performed. If the patient is not seen until the arrhythmia has persisted for more than 48 hours, cardioversion should be postponed until 4 weeks of anticoagulation with warfarin has been accomplished; warfarin should also be continued for 4 weeks after cardioversion.

Treatment of paroxysmal atrial fibrillation or flutter

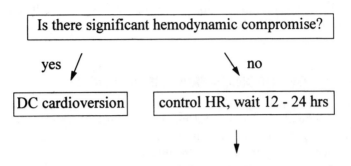

Figure 10.1. In treating paroxysmal atrial fibrillation or atrial flutter, the basic goal is to restore sinus rhythm within 24 hours.

Although acute therapy of paroxysmal atrial fibrillation and flutter is relatively straightforward, chronic management of these arrhythmias can be difficult. The two most difficult questions are whether to administer chronic antiarrhythmic therapy and whether to anticoagulate.

Deciding whether to prescribe antiarrhythmic drugs depends on the frequency and duration of arrhythmias and the associated symptoms. If arrhythmias are infrequent, of short duration, and minimally symptomatic, most experts withhold chronic antiarrhythmic therapy. If arrhythmias are frequent, are longer than 12 to 24 hours in duration, or cause significant symptomatology, chronic antiarrhythmic therapy should be strongly considered. Most patients fall between the two extremes, however, and in most cases a large dose of clinical judgment and a straightforward discussion with the patient regarding the potential advantages and disadvantages of therapy are required before making a decision. If antiarrhythmic therapy is being considered because of severe symptomatology, one can often ameliorate symptoms by having the patient take oral beta blockers or verapamil at the onset of the arrhythmia.

Similarly, the decision whether to anticoagulate must be made more on the basis of clinical judgment than on hard data. Patients with paroxysmal atrial flutter probably do not require anticoagulation. For patients with infrequent episodes of atrial fibrillation lasting only a few hours, especially if the patient is younger than 60 years old, anticoagulation is probably unnecessary. If the frequency and duration of the arrhythmias increase, however, and especially if the patient is older than 60 years, anticoagulation should be strongly considered.

THERAPY OF CHRONIC ATRIAL FIBRILLATION

Chronic atrial flutter is relatively uncommon because most patients with persistent atrial flutter eventually convert to chronic atrial fibrillation. If atrial flutter is persistent, the treatment of choice is to interrupt the reentrant pathways associated with flutter by use of radiofrequency ablation and thereby abolish the arrhythmia.

Chronic atrial fibrillation is defined as atrial fibrillation that has persisted for more than 48 hours. The arbitrary cutoff is chosen because it is generally agreed that after 48 hours, the likelihood of forming atrial thrombi increases greatly—thus, once 48 hours has passed, cardioversion should not be attempted until 4 weeks of anticoagulation has been accomplished.

The decision tree for treating chronic atrial fibrillation is illustrated in Figure 10.2. The fundamental decision that must be made is whether to attempt to restore and maintain sinus rhythm or to merely control the ventricular response. The decision hinges mainly on two considerations: the necessity of restoring the atrial kick and the likelihood of success. If a treatment existed that could maintain sinus rhythm with minimal risk, that treatment would be the clear choice. Maintaining sinus rhythm in a patient presenting with chronic atrial fibrillation, however, is not easy. Without antiarrhythmic therapy, more than 80% of patients relapse within 1 year of cardioversion. Even when antiarrhythmic drugs are used, approximately 50% relapse by the end of 1 year.

Nonetheless, for patients with poor ventricular compliance (i.e., patients with ventricular hypertrophy), the severity of symptoms associated with loss of atrial kick often dictates that aggressive measures be taken to restore sinus rhythm, whatever the likelihood of success. In these patients, after at least 4 weeks of anticoagulation, if possible, sequential trials with antiarrhythmic drugs, including amiodarone, should be tried. With each drug trial, maximal doses should be administered, and if the drug itself does not restore sinus rhythm, DC cardioversion should be performed. If a drug

Treatment of Chronic Atrial Fibrillation

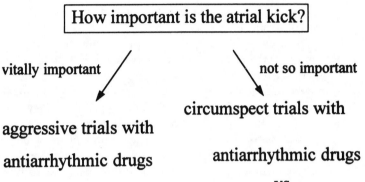

Figure 10.2. In treating chronic atrial fibrillation, the major determination is the importance of restoring and maintaining atrial kick.

proves efficacious, the patient should be encouraged to tolerate mild or moderate degrees of drug toxicity, given the vital nature of the atrial kick. If aggressive trials with antiarrhythmic drugs fail, these are the only patients in whom one should consider radical therapies to maintain sinus rhythm, such as the *maze procedure* (an aggressive open-heart surgical procedure in which the right and left atria are extensively dissected and resewn, in an attempt to eliminate the volume of contiguous tissue necessary to maintain fibrillation). Fortunately, patients with atrial fibrillation in whom restoring sinus rhythm is absolutely necessary are rare.

More commonly in patients presenting with chronic atrial fibrillation, atrial kick is not so vital. In most patients, therefore, attempting to restore and maintain sinus rhythm is an elective procedure. In deciding on a course of action for these patients, the likelihood of success and the risk of drug-induced toxicity should be given much more weight. On average, as noted, the likelihood of success even with antiarrhythmic drug therapy is only approximately 50% at 1 year. A major factor reducing the odds of success is the duration of atrial fibrillation. The longer the patient experienced atrial fibrillation, the lower the odds of maintaining sinus rhythm—after 3 months of atrial fibrillation, the odds of success are very low. The presence of grossly enlarged atria also reduces the chance of maintaining sinus rhythm.

The decision whether to attempt to restore and maintain sinus rhythm is therefore often not straightforward and should be made only after a frank discussion with the patient. Many patients, on hearing about the risks of antiarrhythmic therapy and the moderate odds of success, opt for rate control only, especially if they are only minimally symptomatic from their atrial fibrillation.

Rate control can generally be attained with only moderate difficulty. Most often, digoxin in combination with a beta blocker or verapamil is sufficient, though all three agents are required in approximately 25% of patients. Occasionally, rate control proves very problematic, and radiofrequency ablation of the AV node (with insertion of a permanent pacemaker) needs to be considered. If rate control is chosen, however, rate control *must* be achieved, however difficult it may be—otherwise, rate-related cardiomyopathy may eventually occur. In addition to controlling the rate, serious consideration should be given to chronic anticoagulation. Warfarin (administered to maintain an international normalized ratio of 2.0 to 3.0) decreases the incidence of thromboembolism by 65% to 70% in patients older than 60 years who have lone atrial fibrillation. One aspirin per day reduces the incidence of thromboembolism by 20% to 25%. The benefit of warfarin in younger patients with lone atrial fibrillation is less clear, and aspirin seems a reasonable choice for such patients. In patients older than 75 to 80 years, the risk of bleeding complications with warfarin becomes substantial; whether to use warfarin in these patients remains controversial.

If maintenance of sinus rhythm is elected, drug trials should be conducted much more circumspectly than trials for patients with poor ventricular compliance. After an adequate period of anticoagulation, the patient should be hospitalized and placed on a cardiac monitor for initiation of antiarrhythmic therapy. Selection of an antiarrhythmic drug should be made judiciously; tolerance of the selected drug and avoidance of life-threatening complications should be the primary considerations. If a drug trial fails, the decision to maintain sinus rhythm should be revisited before a second drug trial is undertaken. Quite often, if the patient understands the elective nature of maintaining sinus rhythm, he or she opts out after one or two drug unsuccessful drug trials. Rate control should always be held out as a reasonable therapeutic option.

Treatment of Ventricular Tachyarrhythmias

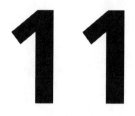

Ventricular tachyarrhythmias are responsible for hundreds of thousands of sudden deaths each year in the United States. Therapeutically, patients at risk for sudden death usually fall into one of two broad categories. First, there are patients who have already experienced an episode of sustained ventricular tachycardia (VT) or ventricular fibrillation. These individuals have already demonstrated a propensity for lethal arrhythmias and are at exceedingly high risk for subsequent sudden death. The second and much larger category consists of individuals who have not yet had sustained ventricular arrhythmias. These patients have underlying cardiac disease accompanied by nonsustained ventricular arrhythmias that are usually asymptomatic. The risk of sudden death for these patients, although demonstrably higher than normal, is generally not as high as that for patients in the first category.

SUSTAINED VENTRICULAR TACHYCARDIA AND VENTRICULAR FIBRILLATION

Patients who have survived an episode of sustained VT or fibrillation have an extraordinarily high risk of experiencing a recurrent arrhythmia. In general, 30% to 50% have a recurrent sustained ventricular tachyarrhythmia within 2 years. Once such an arrhythmia has occurred, aggressive measures must be taken to reduce the subsequent risk of sudden death.

Patients presenting with sustained ventricular tachyarrhythmias do not constitute a heterogeneous group; their individual prognoses can vary significantly. Their risk of dying from recurrent arrhythmias, for instance, is related to the extent of their underlying cardiac disease and to the symptomatology experienced during the presenting arrhythmia. The worse their left ventricular ejection fractions, in general, the higher their risk of recurrent arrhythmias. For years, in fact, it was thought that survivors of cardiac arrest who had relatively normal ventricles had a quite favorable prognosis. Long-term follow-up, however, has revealed that these patients ultimately have a *high* risk of recurrent arrhythmias—it just takes longer for the recurrences to become manifest. Patients who experience loss of consciousness with their presenting arrhythmia have a particularly high probability of dying suddenly with the next episode—the range is 75% to 80%. On the other hand, patients who do not lose consciousness with the initial episode have a low risk of sudden death with the next recurrence—less than 10%. In fact, because the latter group tends to have relatively severe left ventricular dysfunction, they commonly survive several recurrences of sustained VT and die of progressive heart failure.

The heterogeneity of the patient population has significant implications when it comes to measuring the efficacy of any treatment strategy. For instance, because patients with relatively well-tolerated VT often suffer nonarrhythmic death, a treatment that effectively treats their arrhythmias may not measurably prolong their overall survival. On the other hand, the overall survival of patients presenting with ventricular fibrillation and well-preserved ventricular function may not be measurably prolonged by effective antiarrhythmic therapy unless the time of observation is sufficiently long.

Available Treatment Modalities

Four general treatment modalities have been advanced for the management of patients with sustained ventricular tachyarrhythmias: guided drug therapy, empiric drug therapy, implantable defibrillators (ICDs), and ablation of the reentrant circuit. No one modality is suitable for every patient. Optimal therapy must be individualized.

Guided Drug Therapy: The effect of an antiarrhythmic drug on a particular reentrant arrhythmia cannot be predicted. The same drug may have a beneficial effect on one reentrant circuit but a proarrhythmic effect on another. In general, some means must be used to measure the effect of a drug before a patient is committed to long-term therapy. Two general methods of guiding drug therapy have been used in patients with ventricular tachyarrhythmias: Holter monitoring and electrophysiologic (EP) testing.

Holter monitoring was the only methodology available for guiding drug therapy until the late 1970s, and it was widely used until that time. Use of this method requires the presence of ambient ventricular ectopy—either premature ventricular complexes (PVCs) or nonsustained ventricular tachycardia (NSVT)—against which the effect of an antiarrhythmic drug can be measured. A decrease in ectopy is assumed to indicate drug efficacy; an increase in ectopy is assumed to signify potential proarrhythmic potential; no change in ectopy is assumed to mean no effect either way.

Obviously, the success of such a method hinges on an association between the level of ambient ventricular ectopy and the probability of developing a sustained arrhythmia. Unfortunately, no such association has ever been established. In fact, the Cardiac Arrhythmia Suppression Trial (CAST) delivered a death blow to the notion that reducing PVCs also reduces the risk of death. In that trial, significantly reducing ventricular ectopy with Class IC agents was associated with a fourfold *increase* in the risk of sudden death. Simply put, one should not rely on Holter-guided drug selection.

The theory behind EP testing to guide drug therapy is essentially sound. If a reentrant circuit that is capable of generating an arrhythmia exists, all one needs to do to start the arrhythmia is to introduce an appropriately timed electrical impulse into the circuit (see Figure 1.7). This procedure can be accomplished in the EP laboratory by the technique known as *programmed stimulation*, in which a temporary ventricular pacemaker is used to deliver precisely timed, paced impulses into a presumed reentrant circuit. If such a circuit exists and if it has the appropriate EP characteristics (as discussed in Chapter 1), VT can be induced.

EP testing, therefore, can determine whether a reentrant circuit capable of generating a ventricular tachyarrhythmia is present. Among patients presenting with sustained monomorphic VT, the presumed clinical arrhythmia can be induced in approximately 90%. VT can also be induced in 30% to 60% of patients whose presenting arrhythmia is ventricular fibrillation. In addition to assessing the presence or absence of a reentrant circuit, EP testing can be used to assess the effect of an antiarrhythmic drug on the reentrant circuit. The assessment is done by administering a drug and attempting to reinduce the arrhythmia. If a previously inducible arrhythmia is rendered noninducible by a drug, it is assumed the drug has favorably changed the characteristics of the reentrant circuit. Chronic therapy with the drug can then be instituted with a certain level of confidence in its efficacy.

There are many limitations to EP-guided drug selection. For instance, there is no general agreement on which stimulation protocol should be used. This is an important consideration because the more aggressive the stimulation protocol used, the higher the likelihood of inducing an arrhythmia. An aggressive pacing protocol, therefore, yields a higher proportion of inducible arrhythmias—which is good, since therapy can be guided in more patients. However, an aggressive protocol also results in a lower yield of effective drug trials. With the stimulation protocols used in most centers, no more than 30% to 40% of patients tested have had success with any drug in the EP laboratory. The results of serial drug testing in our laboratory are shown in Table 11.1. An additional limitation of EP testing is that interpretation of results is not always straightforward. If the induced arrhythmia is not identical to the patient's clinical arrhythmia or if only a nonsustained arrhythmia can be induced, to what extent can that induced arrhythmia be relied on for serial drug testing? Should a drug that converts a sustained arrhythmia to a nonsustained arrhythmia in the EP laboratory be considered an effective drug? Despite such limitations to EP testing, a multitude of reports from centers around the world have indicated that patients treated with EP-guided drug therapy have had significantly fewer arrhythmias than patients

Table 11.1. Results of Serial Drug Testing for Inducible Ventricular Tachycardia[a]

Drug	No. of Trials	No. Successful	Percentage Successful
Quinidine	155	32	21
Procainamide	198	41	21
Disopyramide	44	6	14
Mexiletine	41	1	2
Phenytoin	221	35	16
Class IC[b]	25	3	12
Combination[c]	51	8	16
TOTAL	759	128	17

[a] Data from Allegheny General Hospital, Pittsburgh, PA.
[b] Flecainide or encainide.
[c] Class IA drug plus mexiletine.

treated empirically. In general, patients treated with drugs selected by EP testing can expect to have a yearly rate of recurrent sustained arrhythmias of approximately 5%, a rate substantially lower than the rate of recurrence generally reported for any other method of selecting drug therapy. Until the early 1990s, EP testing was widely used in patients presenting with sustained ventricular tachyarrhythmias.

There are many reasons EP testing has fallen out of favor in recent years. In the managed care environment, physicians are reluctant to refer patients for testing that is expensive, time-consuming, and effective for only a minority of patients. In addition expectations have been significantly raised by the success of the ICD. Not only is this device highly effective in preventing sudden death, but several reports have indicated that early implantation of an ICD is less expensive than EP-guided therapy. Further, The Electrophysiologic Testing Versus Electrocardiographic Monitoring (ESVEM) trial has called the efficacy of EP-guided therapy into question.

In ESVEM, eligible patients (patients presenting with sustained ventricular arrhythmias who also had both a high degree of ambient ventricular ectopy and inducible VT) were randomized to drug therapy guided either by EP testing or by Holter monitoring. Both groups had similar outcomes. The result has been widely interpreted as indicating that Holter-guided therapy is as effective as EP-guided therapy and that, therefore, EP testing is not necessary in patients with sustained ventricular arrhythmias. Several important criticisms of this study have been leveled, including that only a small minority of patients screened were ultimately enrolled, that a relatively nonaggressive EP protocol was used (so that it was relatively easy to pass a drug trial), and a strong suspicion that covert preselection occurred (i.e., that investigators tended to offer for randomization only patients they suspected would not be significantly harmed by randomization to the Holter arm). However, one does not need to examine the methods of ESVEM in detail to see its major problem; one needs only to look at the published results. In ESVEM, the rate of recurrent arrhythmias for both treatment groups was nearly 40% at 1 year and 66% at 4 years. This recurrence rate, quite simply, is terrible—equivalent to the recurrence rate one would expect to see in patients treated empirically or not treated at all. Thus, the results of ESVEM do not really make the case that EP testing and Holter testing are of equivalent efficacy in treating patients with sustained ventricular arrhythmias;

instead, the results indicate that *neither* the EP testing methodology nor the Holter testing methodology used in ESVEM were useful. Essentially, when selecting drug therapy, one should not use the EP method or Holter method used in ESVEM. Neither method works.

Aside from ESVEM, the long-term results of EP-guided drug therapy has come to be viewed as being less than optimal. A yearly recurrence rate as low as 5% is not negligible—after 5 years, for instance, 25% of patients will have had a recurrent arrhythmia, and many have died suddenly. Unfortunately, evidence exists that there are inherent limits to the efficacy of EP-guided drug therapy, and it is doubtful that results can be improved much beyond this level.

In understanding the inherent limitations to EP testing, one has to discard the widely–held notion that the effect of a drug on a reentrant circuit is an all-or-none phenomenon. Several years ago we conducted a study in which patients who had a successful EP drug trial were subjected to as many as five additional EP trials with the successful drug within 24 hours. We found that, with each repeated trial, a relatively constant proportion of patients (approximately 15%) who had passed every previous trial had inducible VT. In other words, the successful drug was approximately 85% effective during each successive trial (the odds of failing the second trial, for instance, after having passed only one previous trial, was the same as the odds of failing the sixth trial after having passed five previous trials). This result indicates that the effect of a drug on a reentrant circuit is *not* an all-or-none phenomenon. Instead, the inducibility of VT appears to be a probability function, and a successful drug merely reduces the probability that the arrhythmia will be induced with a given level of stimulation.

This notion makes perfect sense when one considers that virtually all complex, multifactorial physiologic processes follow a probabilistic dose-response curve in which a given dose of stimulus yields a certain probability that the target event will occur. Figure 11.1 illustrates a postulated dose-response curve for the inducibility of VT. In this figure, a successful drug trial merely means that the probability curve has been shifted to the right, indicating that a drug defined as being effective in the EP laboratory does not imply absolute protection from recurrent arrhythmias. Perhaps one should consider life itself as representing a chronic, low-grade stimulation protocol—as time passes, the cumulative result of constant low-grade stimulation is a gradually increasing risk of having a recurrent arrhythmia. Therefore, it is probably true that antiarrhythmic drug

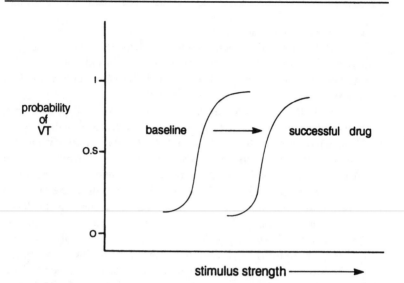

Figure 11.1. For a given stimulus strength (e.g., for a certain number of paced extrastimuli), there is a certain probability that VT will be induced. The relationship between stimulus strength and the probability of inducing VT is presented here as an S-shaped dose-response curve. A successful drug trial shifts the curve to the right; the same stimulus strength is thus associated with a lower probability of inducing VT. As the figure shows, an effective drug does not offer perfect protection from recurrent arrhythmias, it merely reduces the statistical probability of recurrent VT.

therapy, no matter how carefully selected, can never offer absolute protection. All one can hope to do with drug therapy is to move the patient to a more favorable probability curve. (This synthesis might also explain the results of ESVEM—if the EP protocol used is relatively easy to pass, a successful drug trial implies a probability curve that is not shifted very far to the right, and the long-term outcome is predictably less favorable.)

The main question regarding the usefulness of EP-guided drug therapy, then, is not whether it works, but whether it can work well enough. The answer to this question rests on expectations. A 5% per year recurrence rate might look quite favorable compared with other methods of drug selection, but might be completely unacceptable if nonpharmacologic options prove a better outcome.

Empiric Drug Therapy: Using antiarrhythmic drugs empirically means administering them without an attempt to measure their efficacy beforehand. Empiric drug therapy for ventricular arrhythmias was common before 1980 but was deemed unacceptable with the advent of EP testing, especially with the widespread recognition of the phenomenon of proarrhythmia. The empiric use of Class I antiarrhythmic drugs is still universally held to be unacceptable in patients with ventricular tachyarrhythmias. There is support, however, for the empiric use in these patients of one drug—amiodarone.

Amiodarone has traditionally been administered empirically. For years, the empiric use of the drug was justified by the notion that the efficacy of amiodarone, unlike other antiarrhythmic drugs, could not be predicted by EP testing. Later trials indicated that this notion was false. Still, practical considerations almost preclude the use of amiodarone by any means other than empirical ones. The efficacy of amiodarone is not fully manifest until the drug has been administered for a prolonged period—as long as several weeks. If one were inclined to use EP testing to guide therapy with amiodarone, it is unclear how long one should wait before testing. Even more of a problem, if the EP test showed continued inducibility, the patient would have been loaded with a drug that has a half-life of 3 months—one cannot simply discontinue amiodarone and proceed with testing another drug. From a practical standpoint, once a patient has been loaded with amiodarone, the patient has been committed to amiodarone for the foreseeable future.

Further, studies have documented that the empiric use of amiodarone is efficacious in patients presenting with sustained ventricular tachyarrhythmias. The Cardiac Arrest in Seattle—Conventional Versus Amiodarone Drug Evaluation (CASCADE) trial in which survivors of cardiac arrest were randomized to receive either empiric treatment with amiodarone or treatment with conventional drugs guided by EP testing, Holter monitoring, or both, showed that low-dose amiodarone was significantly better than conventional drugs in reducing the incidence of cardiac mortality and recurrent arrhythmic events. Details of how conventional drugs were selected are not provided in the report, but only a small number of patients treated with conventional drugs were clearly drug-responders or nonresponders by EP testing. Further, implantable defibrillators were used in many patients in the study, so the effect of amiodarone in reducing mortality is difficult to evaluate. Yet, CASCADE lends some support to empiric use of amiodarone and has provided justification for ongoing trials comparing empiric use of amiodarone to the ICD in patients presenting with sustained ventricular arrhythmias.

Although empiric use of amiodarone does display efficacy in these patients, its use should be limited. At least one readily identifiable subset, for instance, has a predictably poor outcome with empiric use of amiodarone—patients with inducible VT that is not suppressed during testing with other drugs have a 40% to 50% risk of recurrent arrhythmias within 3 years when they take amiodarone. Further, amiodarone produces a high incidence of long-term, therapy-limiting, and sometimes life-threatening side effects. The incidence of toxicity led even the CASCADE investigators to suggest, in fact, that amiodarone might not be appropriate for patients who were likely to be treated for many years. Empiric therapy with amiodarone should be viewed as reliably shifting the probability curve for recurrent arrhythmias to the right (see Figure 11.1), but the shift is only moderate. Most experts limit the empiric use of amiodarone in patients with sustained ventricular tachyarrhythmias to the subset that has significant underlying disease that renders them poor candidates for an ICD and whose prognosis is judged to be poor regardless of whether they experience a lethal ventricular arrhythmia.

The Implantable Defibrillator: An ICD is a pacemaker-like device that automatically detects the onset of ventricular tachyarrhythmias and automatically terminates them when they occur, either by administering a defibrillating direct current (DC) shock to the heart or by delivering bursts of antitachycardia pacing. The ICD has been in clinical use since the early 1980s, and vast, worldwide experience with the device has been gathered. ICDs can now be implanted with a surgical mortality of less than 1%, and they have proven to be extremely effective in preventing sudden death from ventricular tachyarrhythmias. Survivors of cardiac arrest, whose risk of recurrent life-threatening arrhythmias is otherwise as high as 40% after 2 years, have had the risk of sudden death reduced by the ICD to less than 2% at 1 year and less than 6% at 5 years. No other therapy is as effective in eliminating the risk of sudden death.

The universal acceptance of the ICD has been stalled by its expense and by the argument that, although it unquestionably prevents sudden death, until recently no clinical trial had been conducted to document that it also prolongs overall survival. However, prolongation of overall survival with the ICD is a matter of patient selection—survival is prolonged when it is used in patients who have a high risk of sudden death and whose risk of dying from other causes is relatively low.

Ablation of Reentrant Circuits: Since the reentrant circuits responsible for sustained VT are most often anatomically fixed, disrupting a portion of the circuit with a surgical lesion or by radiofrequency energy delivered by an EP catheter can theoretically "cure" the arrhythmia. Although certain forms of VT have proven highly susceptible to transcatheter ablation (bundle branch reentry and right ventricular outflow tract tachycardia are the least rare examples), in general, only limited success has been achieved in ablating the usual forms of reentrant VT. The ablation of ventricular arrhythmias is an area of active research in many centers, however, and it is likely to become a more widely applicable technique in the next few years.

Overall Approach

Figure 11.2 outlines an overall approach to patients presenting with sustained ventricular tachyarrhythmias. Given the many therapies available for these patients, achieving an optimal outcome strongly depends on choosing the right therapy for the individual patient.

The first and most important step for these patients is assessing and stabilizing any underlying cardiac and metabolic disorders. Underlying heart disease is extremely common in patients with sustained ventricular arrhythmias, and the type and degree of underlying heart disease should be thoroughly evaluated. At minimum, coronary angiography and an assessment of ventricular function should be performed. Coronary disease should be aggressively treated because arrhythmias can be produced by acute (and often occult) ischemic episodes. Anti-ischemic drugs, angioplasty, and bypass surgery should be used as necessary to minimize the chance of recurrent ischemic episodes. Aspirin should be used in most patients with coronary disease, and beta blockers should be administered to patients with previous myocardial infarctions unless strongly contraindicated. Control of lipid abnormalities should be attempted. Therapy of ventricular dysfunction should be optimized and ought to include angiotensin-converting enzyme (ACE)-inhibitors in most patients. Electrolyte disorders should be corrected, especially if the patient is taking diuretics.

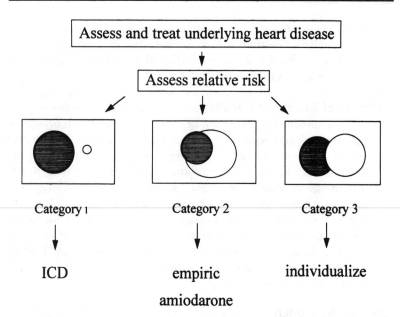

Figure 11.2. Assessment of patients with sustained ventricular tachyarrhythmias. Shaded circles indicate estimated risk of sudden death; open circles indicate estimated risk of death from other causes.

Once the therapy of underlying cardiac disease is optimized, an assessment aimed at judging the relative risk of sudden death from ventricular arrhythmias versus the risk of death from other causes should be performed. Assessment is necessary to make a fundamental decision: Should one use an ICD or should one rely on drug therapy for a particular patient? In making the assessment of relative risks, one should attempt to place the patient into one of three general categories.

Category 1 patients (Figure 11.3) have a relatively high risk of sudden death and a relatively low risk of death from other causes. Survivors of cardiac arrest who have no underlying heart disease or who have heart disease with well-preserved ventricular function most clearly fit this category. These patients have an excellent prognosis as long as sudden death can be prevented. Since an ICD clearly offers the best protection against sudden death, most of these patients should receive it.

Category 2 patients (Figure 11.4) have a relatively high risk of sudden death but also have a high risk of death from other causes—

Category 1

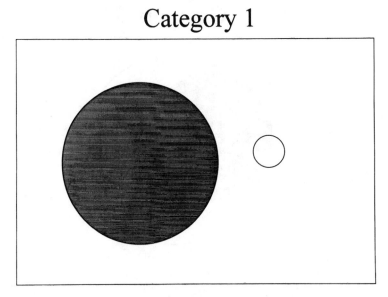

Figure 11.3. Patients in Category 1 have a high risk of sudden death and a low risk of death from other causes. These patients have an excellent prognosis if sudden death can be prevented and are thus optimal candidates for an ICD. Shaded circle indicates estimated risk of sudden death; open circle indicates estimated risk of death from other causes.

most important, the two types of risk overlap, which indicate that even if sudden death is prevented, death is still likely to ensue. The clearest example of a Category 2 patient is the individual with severe, end-stage cardiac disease who is in New York Heart Association (NYHA) Class IV. (Left ventricular ejection fraction, although important, is a less useful indicator of prognosis than is the NYHA class.) An ICD may prevent sudden death in such a patient, but it is very unlikely to substantially prolong survival. In general, one should not submit these patients to the trauma of implanting such a device because they are very unlikely to benefit. Empiric therapy with amiodarone is generally the best option.

Most patients with sustained ventricular tachyarrhythmias fit Category 3 (Figure 11.5). These patients have a moderate to high risk of sudden death, a moderate to high risk of death from other causes, and a moderate overlapping of the risks. A typical Category 3 patient has a moderately depressed left ventricular ejection frac-

Category 2

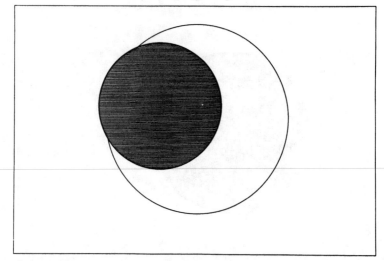

Figure 11.4. Patients in Category 2 have a high risk of sudden death and a high risk of sudden death from other causes with the two kinds of risks overlapping greatly. These patients usually are offered amiodarone as optimal therapy. Shaded circle indicates estimated risk of sudden death; open circle indicates estimated risk of death from other causes.

tion and is in NYHA Class I, II, or III. Therapy for these patients must be individualized. The less severe the underlying heart disease and the worse the presenting arrhythmia (i.e., more hemodynamically unstable VT or ventricular fibrillation), the more likely the patient will benefit from an ICD. The more severe the underlying heart disease (and the higher the risk of non-arrhythmic death), the less likely the patient will benefit from an ICD. Often, EP study is helpful in guiding therapy in these patients.

EP study can be helpful in several ways. Some VTs, as noted, can be ablated using radiofrequency energy delivered via the EP catheter. The two most common ablatable arrhythmias are bundle branch reentry and right ventricular outflow tract tachycardia. Bundle branch reentry has been reported to be responsible for 10% to 15% of VTs occurring in patients with idiopathic dilated cardiomyopathies. Thus, patients with nonischemic cardiomyopathies should usually have a baseline EP study to rule out a

Category 3

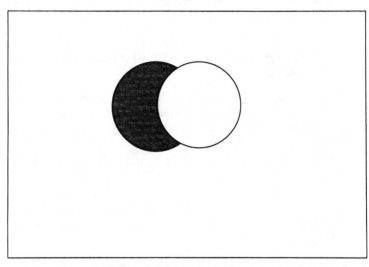

Figure 11.5. Patients in Category 3 have a high risk of sudden death and a high risk of death from other causes, but only moderate overlapping of the risks. Therapy for patients in this category should be individualized. Shaded circle indicates estimated risk of sudden death; open circle indicates risk of death from other causes.

"curable" arrhythmia. Right ventricular outflow tract tachycardias are most often seen in younger patients with no ventricular dysfunction and display a characteristic left bundle branch morphology with an inferior axis. Such a presentation should also prompt EP study. EP-guided serial drug testing is appropriate for some patients, generally those in whom the presenting arrhythmia did not result in loss of consciousness and in whom a 5% per year recurrence of VT is likely to yield a very low risk of sudden death. EP study can also be helpful in prescribing the type of ICD. Patients whose inducible arrhythmias can be terminated by pacing techniques are likely to benefit from a tiered-therapy defibrillator that is capable of pace-terminating slower ventricular tachycardias.

In summary, of all therapeutic modalities available for treating patients with sustained ventricular tachyarrhythmias, no one treatment is suitable for all patients. Treatment must be individualized using a logical, stepwise approach. Such an approach requires care and expertise, but allows suitable therapy to be identified for virtually every patient.

TREATMENT OF NONSUSTAINED VENTRICULAR ARRHYTHMIAS

Appropriately treating patients who have complex ventricular ectopy is inherently more difficult than treating patients who have had sustained ventricular tachyarrhythmias. Patients with complex ectopy are far more numerous than patients with the more severe arrhythmias; their risk of sudden death, although generally more favorable, is also more variable and more difficult to quantify. Treatment, which exposes patients to significant risks and tends to be very expensive, is most often of unclear benefit. Appropriate management, then, depends not only on deciding how to treat, but whether to treat.

Significance of Complex Ventricular Ectopy

The prognostic importance of complex ventricular ectopy (defined by most experts as >10 PVCs/hr during 24 hr of monitoring or the presence of NSVT) depends almost completely on the presence and the extent of underlying cardiac disease. If there is no underlying cardiac disease, complex ventricular ectopy has no prognostic significance at all—the patients have no increased risk of sudden death. However, if patients have underlying cardiac disease with or without complex ventricular ectopy, the risk of sudden death begins to rise. Although complex ectopy alone is not a risk factor, it is relatively uncommon in patients with normal hearts. The presence of unexpected complex ventricular ectopy should thus prompt an evaluation for occult cardiac disease.

One can quantify a patient's risk of sudden death by considering the presence of three separate factors: previous myocardial infarction, depressed left ventricular ejection fraction (i.e., an ejection fraction of less than 0.40), and complex ectopy. The resultant risks are shown in Table 11.2. If previous myocardial infarction or depressed ventricular function are present (as noted, the presence of complex ectopy alone carries no prognostic significance), the 1-year risk of sudden death is approximately 5%. If any two risk factors are present, the 1-year risk of sudden death is approximately 10%. If all three risk factors are present, the 1-year risk is approximately 15%. Thus, patients who have survived myocardial

Table 11.2. Relationship of Ventricular Ectopy to Estimated Risk of Sudden Death

No. of Risk Factors	1-Yr Risk (%)
One	
Previous MI	
LVEF < 0.40	5
Two	
Previous MI + CVE	
LVEF < 0.40 + CVE	10
Previous MI + LVEF < 0.40	
Three	
Previous MI + LVEF < 0.40 + CVE	15

CVE = complex ventricular ectopy; LVEF = left ventricular ejection fraction; MI = myocardial infarction.

infarction or who have depressed ventricular function from any cause have increased risk of sudden death. The risk increases with the presence of complex ventricular ectopy.

Therapeutic Options

Considering that each year 500,000 to 1,000,000 people in the United States have myocardial infarctions, the pool of patients who are at risk for sudden death is huge. From this huge pool of individuals come many of the 400,000 victims of sudden death each year. To make a major impact in reducing the incidence of sudden death, these are the individuals who have to be identified and treated. Unfortunately, none of the potential antiarrhythmic treatments available have been shown to be effective enough to justify exposing all these patients to the risk of therapy or to justify exposing society to the overwhelming expense that would be involved in treating them.

For many years it was assumed that antiarrhythmic therapy aimed at eliminating complex ectopy would ameliorate the risk of sudden death, though there has never been convincing evidence of this assumption. As noted above, CAST most likely placed the final nail in the coffin of antiectopic therapy. In conceptualizing the treatment of complex ectopy itself, the Bear Droppings Theory of Complex Ventricular Ectopy is instructive—if you are walking in the woods and see bear droppings, your chances of being eaten by a bear are higher than if there were no bear droppings. However, if you take out your gun and shoot the bear droppings, you are not reducing your risk. Complex ectopy is best viewed as an indication of increased risk (like bear droppings), not as a target for therapy.

Aside from treating the ectopy itself, two additional treatments have been advanced for reducing the risk of sudden death in these patients: empiric use of amiodarone and the ICD. Of these, prophylactic empiric use of amiodarone has received the most attention. Seven randomized trials have now been completed measuring the effect of empiric use of amiodarone in patients with risk factors for sudden death. The results of the trials are summarized in Table 11.3. Unfortunately, the results do not provide definitive evidence that prophylactic use of amiodarone is helpful. In two trials the Basel Antiarrhythmic Study of Infarct Survival (BASIS) and the Grupo de Estudio de la Sobrevida en la Insuficiencia Cardiaca en Argentina (GESICA), patients treated with amiodarone had improved overall mortality compared with that of control patients. In the Polish Amiodarone Study (PAS), there was an improvement in cardiac mortality with amiodarone, but not in overall mortality. In the Canadian Amiodarone Myocardial Infarction Arrhythmia Trial (CAMIAT) and the European Myocardial Infarct Amiodarone Trial (EMIAT), amiodarone yielded a reduction in arrhythmic death but not in overall mortality. In the Spanish Study on Sudden Death (SSSD) and the Veterans Administration Congestive Heart Failure Antiarrhythmic Trial (CHF-STAT), no improvement in mortality with amiodarone was seen compared with that of controls. Some trials (BASIS, SSSD, and GESICA) suggested a trend toward more benefit in patients with relatively well-preserved ventricular function, and one study (SSSD) appeared to show harm from amiodarone in patients with severely depressed ejection fractions. The fact that in some trials arrhythmic death and cardiac death were reduced but overall mortality was not reduced raises the possibility that amiodarone-related toxicity may have negated any reduction in sudden death. A meta-analysis is planned to try to make better overall sense of these trials, but at present, available evidence does not support the widespread prophylactic use of amiodarone for patients with previous myocardial infarction or depressed left ventricular function.

Several ongoing trials are evaluating the possibility that the ICD may reduce overall mortality in patients at risk for sudden death who have not yet experienced sustained ventricular arrhythmias. The results of one trial, the Multicenter Automatic Defibrillator Implantation Trial (MADIT), were recently made public. In this trial, patients with previous myocardial infarction who had left ventricular ejection fractions less than or equal to 0.35, NSVT, and, during EP testing, inducible sustained VT that was not suppressed by procainamide were randomized to receive either an ICD or conventional drug therapy. MADIT showed an impressive 54% reduction in mortality among patients who received the ICD as compared with patients treated with drugs (80% of whom received amiodarone). Thus, it now seems clear that survivors of myocardial infarction who have NSVT and depressed ventricular function should have EP testing. If patients have induc-

Table 11.3. Clinical Trials Examining the Prophylactic Use of Empiric Amiodarone

Trial	Patient Population	Randomization	Reduction in Arrhythmic or Cardiac Mortality*	Reduction in Total Mortality*
BASIS	MI, CVE	amio 200 mg/day vs. other drugs or placebo	—	Yes
PAS	MI	amio 200 mg/day vs. placebo	Yes	No
SSSD	MI, low EF, CVE	amio 200 mg/day vs. placebo	—	No
GESICA	low EF, CHF	amio 300 mg/day vs. no therapy	—	Yes
CHF-STAT	low EF, CVE	amio 200 mg/day vs. placebo	—	No
CAMIAT	MI, CVE	amio 300 mg/day vs. placebo	Yes	No
EMIAT	MI, low EF	amio 200 mg/day vs. placebo	Yes	No

*Reduction in indicated mortality with amiodarone vs. controls.
BASIS = Basel Antiarrhythmic Study of Infarct Survival; PAS = Polish Amiodarone Study; SSSD = Spanish Study on Sudden Death; GESICA = Grupo de Estudio de la Sobrevida en la Insuficiencia Cardiaca en Argentina; CHF-STAT = Veterans Administration Congestive Heart Failure Antiarrhythmic Trial; AMIAT = Canadian Amiodarone Myocardial Infarction Arrhythmia Trial; EMIAT = European Myocardial Infarct Amiodarone Trial; Amio = amiodarone; CVE = complex ventricular ectopy; EF = left ventricular ejection fraction; MI = myocardial infarction

ible VT that is not suppressible, they should receive an ICD. MADIT is an extremely important study in that, for the first time, it defined a highly effective therapeutic approach to a subset (albeit small) of patients at risk for sudden death. Ongoing trials may add to our ability to treat patients at risk who have not yet had overt sustained ventricular arrhythmias.

Overall Approach

Patients who have underlying cardiac disease and complex ventricular ectopy continue to present a major challenge, both because of the prevalence of this condition and because in most cases there is no clear-cut method of reducing the demonstrably high risk for sudden death. The most important aspect of treating these patients is to aggressively manage their underlying cardiac disease. The

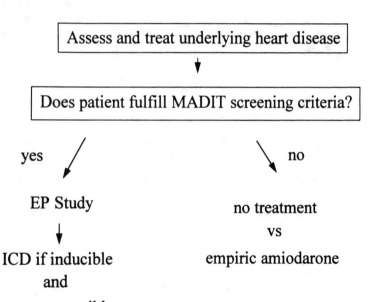

Figure 11.6. Approach to patients with complex ventricular ectopy. A determination should be made as to whether the patient fits MADIT screening criteria. If so, an EP study should be seriously considered; if the patient has inducible VT that is not suppressed during a trial with an antiarrhythmic drug, an ICD should be offered. All other patients should receive no treatment or in some cases, be offered empiric therapy with amiodarone.

approach should be identical to that described for patients presenting with sustained ventricular arrhythmias. The type and extent of underlying disease should be carefully evaluated, and ischemia, heart failure, and lipid abnormalities should be aggressively treated. Therapy specifically aimed at eliminating ventricular ectopy, especially with Class I antiarrhythmic drugs, should be avoided. As noted, it is now clear that the subset of patients with previous myocardial infarctions who have left ventricular ejection fractions less than or equal to 0.35 and NSVT should be referred for EP testing; if the patients have inducible and nonsuppressible VT, they should receive an ICD. Unfortunately, no clear guidelines can be yet stated for using empiric therapy with amiodarone. Although it may be reasonable to use amiodarone in patients with particularly frequent or particularly long episodes of NSVT, no evidence indicates that such patients are at higher risk than those with less frequent or shorter episodes. It may be of some consolation to realize that during the next 3 to 5 years optimal management of this difficult group of patients is likely to become much clearer. Treatment options for these patients are summarized in Figure 11.6.

Index